154

D1498019

A
DIET
FOR
LIVING

JEAN MAYER

Professor of Nutrition,
Harvard University

David McKay Company, Inc.
New York

A Diet for Living

Library of Congress Cataloging in Publication Data

Mayer, Jean.
   A diet for living.

   Includes index.
   I. Nutrition. 2. Diet. I. Title.
TX353.M39   613.2′5   75–11580
ISBN 0–8098–3925–3

MANUFACTURED IN THE UNITED STATES OF AMERICA

To the readers of my magazine articles and newspaper columns. As United States citizens, they have supported through their taxes my laboratory research for the past quarter of a century; through their letters and questions they have inspired me to press for the application of nutritional research to problems of daily life and to try to diffuse practical nutrition knowledge among people everywhere.

FOREWORD

In this book, I have attempted to give answers—short and, I trust, readable—to the most widespread questions that my fellow Americans seem to have about feeding themselves and their families. I have heard or read these questions as a teacher—at Harvard in the School of Public Health, the School of Medicine and the College—as a magazine writer, notably in response to my monthly articles for *Family Health,* and as a biweekly newspaper columnist via the New York Daily News–Chicago Tribune Syndicate. I believe that the information I give here represents what the legal profession calls "the consensus of informed scientific opinion" and can be relied upon by the public.

At the same time, as a research scientist, I know that the most solidly established facts can be successfully challenged by new and imaginative experiments, so that it is possible—indeed, it is likely— that some of the beliefs we now hold will some day be found to be in error. At any given time, however, the prudent person acts on the basis of the best available knowledge.

I also know full well that science, interpreted by common sense, is often more disappointing, and certainly less comforting, than the miracles which the purveyors of nutritional magic can advertise. I live in a world without constant "diet revolutions," where calories do count, where kelp does not necessarily make you beautiful, where a "drinking man's diet" high in fat and alcohol makes you fat, drunk and eventually dead, where "folk medicine" is generally obsolete, a world where real people try to postpone real diseases and keep their family in as healthy a state as they can—within the bounds of the human condition. "The aim of medicine," said Hippocrates, "is to let our patients die young—as late as possible," and in this context, medicine surely includes nutrition.

A single book cannot deal with all aspects of nutrition. Those interested in the details of our knowledge of overweight, in nutrition in disease, in our problems of domestic nutrition policy are referred to previous books. Those interested in problems of worldwide nutrition are invited to wait for a volume now in preparation. This book is about your nutrition in daily life—"a diet for living."

—Jean Mayer

I would like here to gratefully acknowledge the help of my research and editorial assistants, Mr. Harry Wheeler, Mrs. Jeanne Goldberg and Miss Dorothy Campbell and my secretary, Mrs. Arlene Ratner. My publisher, Mr. James Louttit, was very pleasant to work with.

CONTENTS

Contents

3/ The Market and the Kitchen

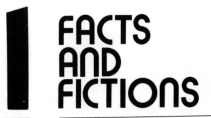

1 FACTS AND FICTIONS

KNOWING
AND
NOT
KNOWING

Nutrition is everyone's cup of tea—with a twist of irony: "facts" everybody "knows" to be absolutely true are precisely those "facts" about which nutritionists are doubtful. On the other hand, some of the facts of which nutritionists are most sure are precisely those that people generally don't accept.

For example, scientists are certain that if you eat more than you need, you gain weight, and if you eat less, you lose weight. Yet the "calories don't count" notion is one of the most persistent *non*facts I've ever run across. No matter how often nutritionists hit it over the head with a club, it gets up again like a cat with not nine but nine hundred lives.

By contrast, scientists are not at all certain about the relationship between brain, emotion, appetite and weight control. For example, it is widely believed some people eat more when they're unhappy. While, by contrast, many people *stop* eating when they are aggrieved. There are firm statements on this subject, but how good is the evidence?

This book is a look at some of the main things nutrition scientists know and don't know about nutrition, and what reasonable course of action we can take, given the current state of our knowledge.

What does the word "nutrition" really mean?

First, let's say what nutrition is not! It is *not* the current craze for massive doses of vitamins, and it is *not* complicated tables of chemical symbols.

It *is* the science that deals with the effects of food on the body. Its roots are not in whim, guesswork, or superstition, or in the personal preferences and private interests of the men and women who practice it. It provides you valuable information on what you can or should eat, how much you should eat, and under what circumstances. And, equally important, what you shouldn't eat, and why.

For instance, a lack of vitamin D causes rickets in children, and an excess of the same vitamin acts as a poison. Omit calcium from your diet, and your bones and teeth suffer. Overeat most animal fats and your blood cholesterol will probably go up.

The guidance presented to you by nutritionists has been gathered, bit by important bit, by trained investigators. Their findings have been checked and confirmed by others equally responsible and—to the advantage of you and your family—professionally challenged by each other.

There is, as you may suspect, much more for nutritionists to learn about this vital subject. But if you learn as much as you can about what is known and apply this information to your daily food selection and food preparation you will stand a far better chance of being around to benefit from the important discoveries about nutrition that are certain to follow.

All of us need to know more about nutrition. We should ask questions of nutritionists and listen to their answers. When the answers are complicated, confusing or unconvincing, we should ask more questions. Believe me, many do! People who have heard me speak on platforms, radio, or television, or have read my books, articles, and columns write to me frequently. They ask important questions, and—when speaking or through my columns in *Family Health* magazine or the *Daily News–Chicago Tribune* Syndicate—I try to provide helpful answers.

If you are typical of most reading and thinking Americans, your first questions will probably be:

Do nutritionists really know very much about energy and weight control?

We know a great deal about these important matters and have known much of it a long time. Since the 1770s we've known you expend (and need) the lowest amount of energy when you're resting at a comfortable temperature, twelve hours after your last meal. Energy requirements increase when you're digesting a meal, when you're exposed to cold, and when you're exercising.

Research over the past two centuries has shown that an adult man may need 1,800 calories per day at rest; 2,400 calories in the course of an ordinary day without much physical activity, and 3,000 calories a day of greater activity (eighteen holes of golf). A trained male athlete practicing hard may expend 3,500 to 5,000 calories. The corresponding figures for women may be 1,500 calories at rest, 2,100 for moderate activity, and 2,600 to 3,500 for great activity. Children need more calories in proportion to their weight. They are growing, very active, and for their size they have relatively more body surface that must be kept warm. Pregnancy and nursing increase requirements by, respectively, 300 and up to 1,000 calories a day if milk production is abundant. Older people require less energy because their metabolism is a little slower and because their activity is decreased.

What is a calorie, anyway? I'm confused about people's caloric allowances. I saw a chart that says my husband should have about 2,500 calories a day but that our teen-age son needs 3,000. Isn't that too much? He weighs thirty pounds less than my husband.

Just to make things clear, let's begin with what a calorie is *not*. It's not a thing. It's a unit of measurement. One calorie (strictly speaking, it should be spelled with a capital C) is equivalent to the amount of energy required to raise the temperature of a liter (about a quart)* of water by 1 degree centigrade. But this energy is used for things other than heating water, of course; our bodies use caloric energy for breathing or moving or keeping warm.

It's likely that your adolescent son does need at least a fifth more calories a day than your husband. Pound for pound, children at all ages need more energy—meaning more calories —and your son needs it, particularly if he's going through a period of rapid growth and great physical activity.

And from where does all this energy come?

Every bit of it is provided by the food you eat: 4 calories per gram from carbohydrates (sugars and starches); 4 calories per gram from proteins; and 9 calories per gram from fats.* If you eat more than you need, you gain weight; if you eat less, you lose weight. (It's that simple.) A pound of fat tissue is equivalent to 3,500 calories. Eat 500 calories per day more than you need and you will gain a pound every week. Eat 500 calories a day less than you require for balance and you will *lose* a pound a week.

Do we know how heredity works to predispose you to overweight?

No. While we know heredity has much to do with whether you are thin or fat, we don't know how it works. We know physical activity thins you down: if you're too inactive, your appetite does not decrease enough and you get fat. But we *don't* know how much heredity influences your spontaneous inclination to exercise or your tendency to get fat when you don't exercise.

In spite of an unfavorable heredity, what can we do?

We do know that if you exercise more and eat less, you will lose weight. We do not know the ideal regimen for weight loss (if indeed there is an ideal regimen). In fact, we are often ineffectual at keeping the weight of patients down after they have reached their target. Patients who respond well to appetite-suppressing drugs appear to be a minority, and physicians have no way of determining in advance which they will be. And, for all the talk of psychosomatic medicine, we know little about

6 *See Appendix I.

the importance of psychological factors in determining weight gain (or weight loss).

All this means one thing: we have to act on the energy balance by eating less and exercising more.

Although in discussions of nutrition we tend to emphasize problems associated with overeating, we must not forget that nutrition involves much more than weight control. For example, consider the questions raised by a pregnant twenty-four-year-old. They are typical of questions frequently asked by readers of my monthly contributions to *Family Health* magazine—and will help introduce us to the questions explored throughout this book.

> *My husband has heart trouble. His fifteen-year-old son lives with us, and I'm expecting my first baby in July. Suddenly, I feel it's terribly important for me to know more about nutrition. But the subject seems so involved. Do I have to learn a lot of details?*

Of course, the more you know about nutrition, the better off you are. But you don't have to memorize long columns of figures or consult a textbook every time you write a shopping list or plan your day's menu. You can start by learning some basic rules, and try to plan ahead so that each meal doesn't become a catch-as-catch-can affair. It's a good idea to have a clear, easy-to-read table of major food groups and nutrients on your kitchen wall. You won't use it like a slide rule; but it will be there to remind you of important foods you may have forgotten to include.

> *I always used to hear about vitamins and minerals; now it's all "nutrients." What's the difference between the terms?*

"Nutrients" is just a short, handy word to describe all the absorbable components of food—carbohydrates, proteins, fats (particularly polyunsaturated fats), vitamins, and minerals—that the body needs in order to fulfill the three main nutritional requirements of good health. Those are: the energy we need to keep warm and to help our organs function, as well as fuel for moving and working; specific nutrients that are needed to utilize foods; and, finally, the nutrients that are required for growth of cells and replacement of used up cells. Besides the carbohydrates, fats, proteins, vitamins, and minerals that should be included, there is one other so essential it is often forgotten—water.

Water doesn't have vitamins, but—depending on its source—it may have some minerals. It may and should contain fluoride, which is good for teeth and bones. But even if it had no "nutrients," it would be still vital to life. Water performs dozens of important functions. If you doubt this, consider that you can live for at least five weeks without food, but only one week without water.

Fiber (roughage), though not "nutritive," is also important for good health.

Does our son need any special nutrients that my husband and I don't need? And now that I'm expecting a baby, what about me? Do I need more nutrients?

Both boys and girls, because they are growing, need more proportionately of most nutrients than do adults. For example, they need more calcium to build bones and more iron to manufacture new blood. Teen-age girls, in particular, need more iron because of menstrual losses, which can be considerable.

You, as an expectant mother, need more calories than you usually do, and much more calcium, and more of all the vitamins and minerals. And if you're planning to nurse your baby, as I hope you are, keep in mind that a nursing mother uses up some 800 to 1,000 calories a day just making milk. You should also drink plenty of milk for calcium.

In addition to wanting to nurse my baby, I hope to keep my figure. Can I drink skim milk instead of whole milk? And is it true that if I don't get enough calcium while I'm pregnant, the baby will rob me of it, harming my teeth as a result?

As long as the skim milk you drink is vitamin D–enriched or you get vitamin D elsewhere, you can drink it rather than whole milk. So can everyone else in a family, with the exception of small babies, for whom a pediatrician's advice should be sought. If you don't have enough calcium in your diet, the growing fetus will indeed get calcium, from your bones if not from your teeth. This would be even more dangerous if you attempted to breast-feed without getting sufficient calcium from milk and cheese.

Why are bread and other grain products enriched with nutrients?

This is done because the added nutrients are those most likely to be missing from your diet if it isn't well balanced. Most of us get more than enough protein, but many of us get only borderline amounts of iron. Other nutrients, such as vitamin B_1, are added because they were lost in the milling of the grain. Niacin is added to corn because many people who eat a lot of corn but little meat are in danger of pellagra from lack of niacin and the amino acid tryptophan. The body can make niacin from tryptophan, which is low in the type of protein found in corn. Whole grain bread or bread made from "undermilled flour" (off-white bread) contains all these nutrients and, in addition, bran (or fiber), useful for more rapid elimination of fecal material. By shortening the time feces stay in the intestine, fiber may also protect us from risks of diverticulitis and cancer of the large bowel, the second most frequent malignancy in women as well as in men.

Is there any way I can be sure we're getting all the nutrients we need? Can you outline an ideal diet?

I could, but I won't. The certain way to get all the nutrients you need is to get variety. Try all kinds of foods, except those you have been advised to avoid. Don't get into food ruts; vary your menu from day to day. Don't exclude whole classes of foods, such as potatoes and bread, which some people unwisely eliminate when they're on weight-reduction programs. Do cut down on the amount of sugar and salt in your diet.

A specific diet, with each day's food tabulated, cannot and should not be prescribed as the model for a healthy person, particularly when variety is a desirable goal. Fortunately, it isn't necessary. You can insure good nutrition if you eat, every day, at least one and preferably several servings from each of the seven major groups: (1) green, yellow and leafy vegetables; (2) citrus fruits, tomatoes, raw cabbage and salad greens; (3) potatoes, other vegetables not included in group (1), and non-citrus fruits; (4) milk and milk products; (5) meat, poultry, fish, eggs, dried beans and peas, and nuts; (6) bread, flour and cereals; and (7) some butter and fortified margarine. (Using one of the "soft," polyunsaturated margarines may be useful, unless you *know* that your cholesterol is low. Your intake of eggs should be restricted to two or three a week, as recommended by the American Heart Association.)

That sounds like a seven-course menu for every meal. Won't it add up to too many calories?

Here's a one-day menu that covers the whole thing: orange juice and cereal with milk and sliced bananas for breakfast; a tuna fish salad sandwich (with lettuce), fruit cup, and milk or fruit juice for lunch; pea soup, chicken, tossed green salad, baked potato with a little margarine, fruit juice or milk, and ice cream for dinner. Grown-ups can skip the ice cream and have fruit or low-fat cheese for dessert. This typical menu needn't add up to an excess of calories. The secret is that you don't have to eat a *lot* of any of those things. Many people have the mistaken notion that "diet" means the *kind* of food they consume, not the *amount*. But the plain fact—*the most important fact of all*—is that two ounces of steak contain exactly half the calories of four ounces, and four ounces contain half as many as eight. This is true of any food—from steak to chocolate pie. Eat plenty of *different* foods—*but watch the size of those portions!*

Is orange juice the only way to get vitamin C?

No, and most of the other sources have fewer calories. Try lemons, limes, green pepper, grapefruit, fresh strawberries, crisp salad greens, and that great low-calorie beverage—tomato juice. Don't forget raw cabbage. Baked or boiled potatoes in sufficient amounts are also a good source of vitamin C.

How much milk does a child need? Does an adult need any?

Milk and cheese are valuable sources of calcium, vitamin A, high-quality protein and other nutrients. A child should have from three to four cups of milk a day, an adult two cups. Milk haters can eat cheese; weight watchers can try skim milk. But skim milk doesn't have the vitamin A or vitamin D of whole milk, unless it's fortified. (Fortification is the addition of

10

nutrients not originally in a food. Enrichment restores the nutrients eliminated during processing.)

If you eat a lot of fish and chicken, do you need red meat?
Red meat is not at all mandatory. Fish and chicken are excellent sources of good-quality protein. And they have two advantages over red meat: they're generally lower in calories and fat, and what fat they have is less saturated. I recommend that children, women of childbearing age, and pregnant women eat kidney, liver, heart and other variety meats for the iron and vitamins they contain. Don't forget that dried peas and beans, lentils, soybeans, nuts, and peanut butter are good sources of protein. An all-vegetable diet that is rich in these foods can be quite adequate in protein, though it may be low in iron and calcium and deficient in vitamin B_{12} and D.

Are eggs necessary?
They are certainly useful. Eggs are an excellent source of protein and a variety of other nutrients. Children should eat them, and they are good for young women. Again, adult men and older women (after the menopause) should eat eggs rarely, unless their blood-cholesterol level is low (under 220) and is tested regularly. Egg yolks are very high in cholesterol.

I read that a leading Russian nutrition expert advocates four meals a day to keep up the accelerated pace of daily living. Is this a good idea?
This hardly is a revolutionary concept. The late-evening snack suggested for Russians has been, for better or for worse, an intrinsic part of the American way of life. Indeed, the average American, whose days are long and whose dinner hour tends to be much earlier than that of his European counterpart, can become quite hungry by 10:00 P.M. For him the evening snack is a usual thing.

The important issue is not how many times a day you eat, but—when you add up the quantity consumed—what is your nutritional record? Has your diet been adequate? Is the distribution of your calories throughout the day such that you burn up as many calories as you take in?

11   There is nothing intrinsically wrong with four, five or even

six meals a day. Many dieters, in fact, prefer to spread out their caloric allowance this way. As long as the total caloric intake is what you need—and no more—it's okay. But countless trips to the kitchen for evening nibbles can become dangerous.

What conclusion should I draw from what nutritionists know and don't know about what to eat and what not to eat?

You—and we nutritionists, too—have to look askance at too rapid a rate of change in the nature of our food supply. The trend toward constantly increased use of refined flour, sugar, isolated single proteins, and purified oils and fats may go beyond our capability to know what nutrients to replace by enrichment and fortification. The only safe course is to continue to make sure that a large proportion of our diet consists of a *variety* of whole-grain products, fruits and vegetables, animal products and—for young women and children—eggs.

You constantly urge people to learn more about nutrition and to apply in their eating habits the learning they acquire. Have you personally made any changes in what you eat and don't eat as a result of current findings in nutrition?

I have made some changes because I believe the world has rarely been more interesting than it is right now. I suspect that in the approaching future it will be even more interesting, and I want to be around long enough to find out how a lot of fascinating things now going on turn out.

So I must not include in my diet anything that has even a tiny chance of contributing to my early demise; nor must I leave out of it anything that might help postpone that grim event. I no longer drink much whole milk. I have given up butter (this is a real sacrifice because I do not like and therefore do not use margarine). Only infrequently, no oftener than once a week, do I eat one or at most two eggs. It is years now since I have touched bacon. And seldom do I sprinkle salt on anything. But I'm still left with an abundance of excellent things to eat. Many of them taste good, too. Fish, turkey, whole-grain cereals, fruits, vegetables, for example, are foods I very much enjoy.

2 THE ABC'S OF PROTEINS

For many people, protein has taken on an aura of the "super-food," representing the best of foods' nutrients—the body builder, the muscle maker and the weight reducer. Americans tend to equate the word "protein" with beef, considering chicken, milk, fish, or cheese as poor "also rans," and vegetables and bread as utterly devoid of the magic stuff. Protein, it is widely believed, contains no calories. In fact, it is thought that protein "burns up fat," so the more protein you eat, the thinner you will get!

Proteins (plural because there are more than one) do deserve their reputation of being marvelous substances. They are the most complex substances known to man. One scientist has called them "the noblest pieces of architecture invented by nature." But, unfortunately, most of proteins' current reputation is based on a muddle of mistaken myths.

Just what are proteins?

Let me draw an analogy. Back in 1454 Gutenberg invented movable type. Instead of having to make each letter individually in each word of each sentence—as you would carve your name on a tree—he made molds from which he could produce in metal dozens of copies of each letter. These could be dropped into place to print anything of any length: short poems and long ones, plays, novels, histories, recipes, encyclopedias, newspapers, magazines and so on. Proteins are formed on the same principle. Proteins, which can be likened to words and sentences, are made up of twenty amino acids, many used more than once, comparable to the twenty-six letters of varying combinations of our alphabet. And from these twenty amino acids, millions of different proteins can be manufactured.

What do all these proteins do?

Each type of cell in every animal, vegetable and microbe contains its own particular kind of proteins. Thousands of them. Indeed, proteins are the primary, basic components of life (hence their name, which comes from a Greek word meaning "of first rank"). Some proteins, such as the protein in bones, are part of the carpentry that keeps us erect. Some glue our cells together. Some (enzymes) act as chemical engineers whose job is to help put other substances together or take them apart, while others (antibodies) protect us from disease as part of our immune mechanism.

Can nutritionists speak more confidently about their knowledge of protein? Does protein really build muscle?

Fortunately, they can. We have known for at least a century and a half that you need food containing nitrogen. Little by little, we have discovered the structure of proteins, those building stones called amino acids. Some of these (the "essential" amino acids) have to be provided in the diet because the body cannot make them, while others (the "nonessential" amino acids) under the right conditions can be synthesized in the body. For a century we've known that all proteins are not equivalent. For example, gelatin is a source of proteins, but you couldn't live on it as your *only* source because the proteins in it are *incomplete*. Incomplete proteins are somewhat, or completely, lacking in certain essential amino acids. In general, animal proteins (eggs, milk, meat and fish) are complete proteins, while vegetable proteins are often incomplete. This means animal proteins contain the twenty amino acids that make up protein in about the same proportions we need to make body protein. Vegetable proteins have amino acids in less favorable proportions.

A mixture of animal and vegetable proteins adds up to better nutrition than do vegetable proteins alone. In fact, a mixture of vegetable proteins—say rice and peas—together with a relatively small amount of animal protein (as in a Chinese meal) may be as good as animal protein, considerably less expensive, and lower in fat than a huge steak!

In one sense, protein builds muscles. Protein is second only to water as a main constituent of body structures, particularly muscles but also tendons, skin, and other tissues. We need protein to develop muscles and keep them healthy. But muscle "building" or firming and strengthening doesn't come from eating an unusually large amount of protein. Muscle building takes exercise. And exercise does *not* increase the need for protein over and above what your body requires if you lead a sedentary life.

If each animal and vegetable has its own characteristic proteins, how can humans live on proteins from other animals or plants?

These proteins are broken up by stomach acids and enzymes into fragments, and in the intestine they are broken down even further into single amino acids. Then they're reassembled into human proteins.

The body can even make some of its own amino acids out of other amino acids. These are the "nonessential" amino acids —so called not because they aren't essential to life, but because it isn't essential to eat these specific amino acids to get them. So long as you eat enough protein generally your body can manufacture them. Eight of the amino acids are essential; they must come from food because the body can't make them from other substances.

You need some kinds of protein more than others. We can still use our analogy with printing: In the English language the most frequently used letter is *e;* the next is *t.* So you need more of these letters to write something in English than you need g's or x's. Thus, proteins that contain the right proportion of amino acids necessary for life and health are obviously better for you, or, as scientists say, have greater "biological value."

The value of breast milk is high—close to a perfect 100. Whole-egg protein is a close second—about 94—while cow's milk ranks 85 and meat and fish are fourth on the list, ranging from 76 to 86. Rice (surprisingly) ranks a fairly good 80. Lesser values are found in potatoes, soybeans, grains, peas and beans.*

In case you still aren't convinced that protein is more than such a simple affair as a hunk of beefsteak, let me add that a particular protein not only contains many different kinds of amino acids but lots of little "bits" of each one, arranged in different places in its structure. A molecule of a simple little protein in your blood called "serum albumin" contains 526 amino acids of 18 different kinds!

Does meat contain all the proteins we need to stay healthy?

You already know that meat ranks a little lower than some other proteins in value. But there's more to it than that. For one thing, about 60 percent of the calories in meat come from fat; hence you have to eat a lot of calories and a lot of saturated fats to get the proteins from beef. Not only that, a mixture of proteins is often better than a single one—or several single ones —taken one at a time. Wheat, for example, is low in the amino acid lysine. But milk does contain it more liberally. So—believe it or not—ordinary white bread made of wheat and skim-milk powder is a fairly good source of protein with good biological value.

Chinese meals show how well proteins supplement each other. Rice is low in four essential amino acids, but two of these are supplied by beans, and the other two are in beef, pork, poultry or fish, the usual components of Chinese dinners.

How much protein do I have to eat?

Convincing studies have shown that an ounce a day of pure protein of good quality is minimally sufficient for the average adult woman. A man, being bigger, needs somewhat more. Children, adolescents and pregnant and nursing women need considerably more. A number of experiments have shown that habitual strenuous exercise does *not* increase protein requirements, in spite of almost universal belief to the contrary among coaches, athletes and the public.

If protein is as important as nutritionists say it is, wouldn't we be better off eating more?

We don't know the advantages, if any, of going far above the minimum protein necessary for life or optimal growth. In the adult, we have seen that an ounce or so of a good protein daily will maintain the average man or woman in good health. To ensure a safety margin, the usual recommendation is about two ounces. Actually, many American men eat between three and four ounces of protein every day, three to four times as much as is required, and almost twice the recommended allowance, which already has a margin of safety.

While both low-protein and high-protein diets have had their proponents, the evidence in favor of or against either position is scanty. The long-term differences between high- and low-protein diets are especially hard to evaluate. High-protein diets are usually based on meat and are high in saturated fats (beef may have up to three times as many calories from fat as from protein). Very low protein diets are often poor from other viewpoints; for instance, they are low in vitamins and minerals.

Do athletes or other active people need more protein than sedentary types?

No. Protein needs depend first on size. Generally, the larger you are the more protein you need. Then there's growth: pound for pound, children need more than adults, and infants need the most. Pregnant women and nursing mothers also need extra protein. An average 130-pound woman needs a minimum of one ounce of the best-quality protein. In practice she will do very well with about two ounces of animal and vegetable protein (half and half is an easy rule of thumb), and a lean 190-pound man will do very well with three ounces.

Although the body does "turn over" protein and needs regular replacements, it doesn't turn it over a bit faster whether you're an Olympic swimmer or just an ordinary citizen who sits and watches the Olympics on TV. Swiss scientists proved this a century ago by studying mountain climbers, and it's been proved again innumerable times since. Nevertheless, coaches and players continue to believe that large amounts of steak improve physical prowess. So a great many young men and women are getting into the habit of eating what passes for a high-protein diet that is actually loaded with saturated fats and cholesterol and may lead to coronary disaster in middle age.

One often hears nutritionists glibly refer to the "necessary" intake of proteins as somewhere between 50 to 60 grams a day. How can you tell if you're getting 60 grams of protein a day?

Making a rough estimate of your protein intake is fairly simple. An ounce of relatively lean meat, or an ounce of fish, poultry or cheese contains, on the average, 7 grams of protein, as does one egg. Fattier meats, of course, provide less. An 8-ounce glass of milk provides 8 grams. A serving from the bread and cereal group contains about 2 grams, and a cup of dried peas or beans is about 14 grams or about twice the amount in an ounce of meat.

So, if you eat 6 ounces of meat-group foods (which adds up to 42 grams of protein), 2 cups of milk (16 grams) and 4 servings from the bread-and-cereal group (8 grams), you have easily met your protein requirement for the day.

Cereal proteins, which are not as complete as others, are enhanced by combining them with animal proteins. Eating dry cereal with milk is a classic example of how cereal protein is improved in a natural combination of foods. Protein is one of the nutrients listed in grams per serving right on the label under the guidelines for nutritional labeling of foods.

Is protein nonfattening?

That's the most persistent protein myth of all, and furthest removed from fact. Protein contains 4 calories per gram— exactly the same as starch or any other carbohydrate. In fact, only 27 percent of the calories in the average beefsteak are proteins. We need proteins for health, and the backyard barbecue wouldn't be the same without them. But calories are calories, no matter where you find them. Enjoy your meat, make sure you get many kinds of protein for your health's sake, but don't count on proteins to make you slim or give you longer nails and silkier hair or work similar wonders. Not even protein can perform such miracles.

A friend is taking protein wafers as a dietary supplement because he's concerned that he doesn't get enough protein. He suggested that I do the same. What are protein wafers? Are they a good nutritional supplement?

Trying to increase protein intake with protein wafers is like filling a bathtub with a thimble. It will take a long time to get anywhere, and at what a cost!

Protein wafers are made from combinations of soy protein, malt extract for flavoring and a bit of dried-milk powder. Examining samples at a local drugstore, I found that nine tablets, the amount suggested for daily consumption, would yield a little over 2 grams of protein and cost between 13 and 18 cents, depending on the brand.

You can purchase enough nonfat dried milk (incidentally, the best-quality protein in these wafers, but present in the smallest amount) to make a whole quart of milk. That milk would contain sixteen times as much protein, as well as many other essential nutrients, for just about the same amount of money as the wafers cost.

In order to get the same amount of protein as in an ounce of sirloin steak, you'd need to crunch down twenty-seven wafers, costing, at this writing, many times the price of the steak. Protein wafers cannot be seriously regarded as an efficient dietary supplement.

Are the quality and cost of meat related only to taste, or do they have anything to do with nutrition? Do very inexpensive steaks have the same nutrition as prime ribs in a good restaurant?

The quality of the protein is the same. In fact, cheap cuts such as liver, heart and other organ meats have much more protein in them and much less fat. They are real nutritional bargains. The only problem is that you may have to acquire a taste for them, and they take more time and skill to prepare than a sirloin. Paradoxically, very expensive steaks in restaurants are usually well-marbled with fat, so they actually have less protein per pound than cheaper cuts.

If you eat a well-balanced diet but take in more protein than you need, does your body store it or is it simply wasted?

Assuming you are in good nutritional health and have been eating an adequate diet all along, excess proteins are, in a sense, wasted. That is, the body does not use them as proteins. They are broken down, or "de-aminized," and used for energy. If the body does not need them for that purpose, they are stored as fat.

Protein foods generally cost more than carbohydrates and fats, so that's a pretty expensive way to get your energy. Since, gram for gram, protein supplies as many calories as carbohydrates, a diet high in protein is of no particular advantage in a weight-reduction program.

Beyond meeting the daily needs for growth and repair of body tissue, there is just no good reason for an extraordinarily large protein intake, despite all the claims of advocates of high-protein diets.

Why do people need to eat meat? After all, many animals that are well-muscled don't seem to need protein. They live on grass and hay or things like that.

Yes, they do, but there's a big difference in the way their stomachs work. Many animals, unlike people, make their own protein. For instance, a bull, which certainly is a most muscular animal, has four stomachs which contain as much as 100 pounds of protein-providing bacteria. The bacteria live on the hay, the bull lives on the protein from the bacteria. Man's single stomach can't produce enough protein, so people have to eat foods that supply it. But, as we shall see, man's protein does not have to come from meat alone.

3 FACTS ABOUT FATS

Fats (and oils, which are fats that are liquid at room temperature) add up to one of the main sources of energy in the American diet.

Fats and oils are sometimes divided into visible and invisible fats. The visible are those we add to foods: butter, shortenings, and corn, peanut and other cooking or salad oils. The invisible, those already contained in food, include: the butterfat in whole milk, the fats in eggs, fish, meats, nuts and other things we eat.

Fat makes our food more palatable than it would otherwise be and also contributes to the "had enough" feeling. It supplies essential fatty acids. It provides transport for the fat-soluble vitamins. It offers calories in compact form. It travels around the body through the bloodstream. And it confuses people who ask me such questions about it as I shall now attempt to answer:

What are fats made of?

The main components of fats in food and in the body are various fatty acids. Butter, for instance, contains more than twenty-nine kinds. The difference of taste in fats depends upon which fatty acids predominate. The distribution of fatty acids also dictates the temperature at which a fat melts—and thus determines whether fats are solid or liquid at room temperature. It makes little or no difference to the number of calories per gram: all fats and oils contain approximately 9 calories per gram.

What are fatty acids?

Fatty acids are chiefly carbon atoms arranged in a straight chain, with the acid part on one end. All along the carbon chain are little arms sticking out. What is on the arms is what counts and what determines whether the fatty acid is saturated, monounsaturated or polyunsaturated.

What are saturated fatty acids?

Saturated fatty acids have hydrogen stuck on all the little arms; they are "saturated" with it. This type is the chief component in animal (meat) fats, butter and dairy products. Such fats do not melt at room temperature. Palmitic, stearic and myristic acids are saturated fatty acids. They raise the level of cholesterol in the blood.

What are unsaturated fatty acids?

Two of the arms of unsaturated fatty acids have no hydrogen. Instead, they hold hands. So the fatty acid is not fully filled, not saturated with hydrogen. The most common monounsaturated acid is oleic. Olive and peanut oils contain this type of fatty acid predominantly. They neither raise nor lower blood cholesterol.

What are polyunsaturated fatty acids?

Two or more pairs of the arms of polyunsaturated fatty acids hold hands and have no hydrogen ("poly" means "many"). The least saturated fats, they are the major type found in corn, soybean, cottonseed and, particularly, safflower oils. Polyunsaturated fatty acids cannot be synthesized in the human body. These fatty acids are liquid at room temperature and tend to lower the blood cholesterol.

How are the fatty acids arranged in fats and oils?

22 Groups of three fatty acids are combined with a short molecule of glycerol (more popularly known as glycerin), pretty much as the long tines of a fork are hooked together by being stuck on a short base. A better comparison would be with a three-toothed Spanish-type haircomb.

Is cholesterol also a fatty acid?

No. Cholesterol is a more complicated substance, much more like a wax than like an ordinary fat. The body requires it. It is present in the walls of all cells. Some hormones and vitamin D are made from it. Cholesterol is manufactured, in at least the required amount, by the body, regardless of the amount in the diet. A high dietary intake depresses the body synthesis of cholesterol, but not enough to cancel out the effect of the diet. A high saturated fat intake also tends to increase the amount of cholesterol circulating in the blood. When the blood has too much cholesterol, whether manufactured by the body (heredity is a factor here) or stimulated by a high fat diet or from the ingestion of cholesterol itself (egg yolk is one of the chief food sources), cholesterol settles in the walls of blood vessels. They become less elastic (hardening of the arteries, or atherosclerosis), and grow narrow so that blood flow is slowed or even stopped. If this happens in a major heart or brain artery, the result is a coronary or a stroke.

What is hydrogenated fat?

Hydrogenated fat is simply unsaturated fat that has had hydrogen added to it, filling up the empty arms on the carbon chain. The more fats are hydrogenated, the harder they are and the better they keep, but the more they raise the blood-cholesterol level and the more they endanger your heart's health.

Is weight loss always accompanied by a lowering of blood cholesterol?

Sometimes the carrying out of a successful weight-reduction program brings with it a lowering of blood cholesterol. Sometimes it doesn't. Often someone loses unwanted pounds and simultaneously his blood cholesterol drops, only to return to its former heights shortly thereafter. An obesity-fighter may go on a high-saturated fat diet (masquerading as a low-carbohydrate one) and rid himself of unwanted weight without lowering the blood cholesterol; he may, indeed, actually increase it.

What kind of fat is the fat in fish: unsaturated, saturated or polyunsaturated? And how does fish shape up as a source of nutrients?

Fish fat is high in polyunsaturated fat, low in saturated fat. Mackerel and halibut are particularly good sources of polyunsaturates. In sardines canned in cottonseed oil—but not those in peanut oil or olive oil—the polyunsaturated oil adds its effect to that of the fish.

At a time when mortality from heart disease is overwhelmingly our Number One health problem, one of the most important health measures any adult man (or postmenopausal woman) can adopt is to replace beef by fish at least three times a week. Eating fish cakes, fish balls, or fish sticks is an easy, convenient method of carrying out this resolution. Choose, if possible, those prepared with polyunsaturated fats.

Fish is an excellent source of a number of nutrients, particularly protein (about 25 percent of the weight of fish and almost 100 percent of the dry weight of a lean fish like cod). Fish fillets are solid blocks of excellent quality protein.

Fish—particularly small fish whose bones are eaten—provide calcium (4 ounces of sardines cover a day's recommended dietary allowance of calcium). They also contain fluorine; that lowly canned sardine is an excellent source of this tooth-protecting trace element, especially important for children living in communities where the water is inadequately supplied with fluorine.

Fish contains pyridoxine, an important B vitamin, and is particularly rich in the amino acid lysine. Fish is also a satisfactory source of thiamine and riboflavin, two vitamins that nicely survive industrial processing. In a sardine or tuna fish sandwich, the building blocks of the fish protein complement those of the bread protein, so that the biological value of the sandwich protein is greater than the sum of its parts.

Are we eating just about the right amount of fat or too much or too little?

Since 1900 the percentage of calories represented by fat in the diet has inched upward from about 30 percent to well over 40 percent (about 43 percent is the latest figure). In certain groups, such as male college students and businessmen, it exceeds 50 percent. It used to be taught that the replacement of starches by fats, calorie for calorie, was a matter of no consequence. The pioneer work of Ancel Keys, shortly after World War II, suggested that a high-fat intake might be associated with a greater prevalence of heart disease. During the past twenty years, evidence has accumulated indicating that elevated levels of cholesterol in the blood—from large amounts of saturated fat in the diet—were accompanied by an increase in cardiovascular disease.

By contrast, it appears that polyunsaturated fats decrease the level of blood cholesterol. There is some evidence—some of it obtained in my laboratory—that prolonged daily exercise seems to decrease blood cholesterol. Uncorrected high blood pressure, overweight, the presence or absence of certain trace minerals, stress, lack of sleep, cigarette smoking, and for its victim, diabetes, may promote heart attacks and strokes. It appears to be the better part of wisdom to try to keep cholesterol in our blood down by reducing total fat, saturated fat and cholesterol in our diet.

Do we really need fats? Couldn't we cut them out of our diet entirely if we want to lose weight?

In the first place, to cut all fats from your diet, you would have to stop eating meat, eggs, fish, nuts and dozens of other nutritionally useful and tasty foods. You would probably find it difficult to cook without any shortening or oil. Fats are a major source of energy, and many fats provide other important nutrients. Butter and fortified margarine, for instance, give us vitally needed vitamin A; vegetable oils contain vitamin E, and meat, fish, eggs and nuts supply protein as well as plenty of necessary vitamins and minerals. Last, but not least, many fats contain polyunsaturated fatty acids, which are indispensable to life. This is particularly true of most vegetable oils, notably corn oil, safflower oil, soybean oil, and also fish liver oil and most fish fats.*

Why do we keep hearing that we should cut down on fats? And how can I tell whether I'm eating saturated or unsaturated fat?

25   *See Appendix III.

It's not only the amount of fat we consume that is so important, but the *kind*. (Futhermore, a high-fat diet also means a high-calorie diet, which is a matter of concern if you have a weight problem.) Many nutritionists and physicians attempt to persuade people to reduce the *saturated* fats in the diet, since saturated fats raise cholesterol in the blood.

Most meat and animal fats—including the butter fat of milk and cheese, and the fat of eggs—are saturated. Beans, corn, nuts, and fish contain unsaturated and polyunsaturated fats. When it comes to cooking fats and salad oil, look at the label. Hydrogenated fats are preponderantly saturated; pure vegetable oils are not. An exception is coconut oil, a saturated oil found in a good many convenience foods and coffee whiteners. Olive oil is mostly mono-unsaturated rather than polyunsaturated, and is therefore less useful. The obvious difference between saturated and unsaturated fats is that the former remain solid at room temperature.

4 ... AND ABOUT CARBOHYDRATES

Carbohydrates—made of carbon and of hydrogen and oxygen in the proportion seen in water, hence their name—are major sources of energy for most of the world's people. They are assembled in green plants by the light from the sun working on carbon dioxide and water. They come to us as starches and sugars for nourishment and as cellulose for roughage ("fiber").

Usually carbohydrates are the principal suppliers of the body's energy. In the United States they constitute about 45 percent of the caloric intake, whereas in poorer lands the figure may rise to 80 percent. The starches figure prominently in such foods as potatoes, cereals and breads. Ordinary table sugar, white or brown, is sucrose, made of fructose and glucose, two "simple" sugars. When utilized by the body, 1 gram of carbohydrate yields 4 calories, as does 1 gram of protein. (One gram of fat, remember, yields 9 calories.)

Glucose (known also as dextrose, grape sugar—or blood sugar) deserves emphasis. It can be synthesized by the body from other carbohydrates and also from protein. Glucose is the only true "brain food." It is overwhelmingly the main fuel for the brain (perhaps the only one under normal circumstances).

The main sugar in milk is lactose. Eighty percent of the calories in the bread we eat comes from carbohydrates.*

What is the value of the "carbohydrate-free" diet?

None. Starches and sugars (carbohydrates) contain roughly 4 calories per gram, the exact figure for protein, which many people consider "low-cal," if not "calorie-free." Carbohydrates, as I just explained, appear to be the near-exclusive fuel of our brain. Eating a carbohydrate-free diet (or less than 400 calories of carbohydrates per day) means that we have to convert protein into carbohydrates, thus robbing the body of protein.

I understand the need for carbohydrate to provide glucose. Are all carbohydrates then equivalent? Can I take mine as table sugar?

I'd rather you wouldn't. We know that ordinary sugar is highly destructive to teeth. Moreover, there is unconfirmed evidence that eating large amounts of sugar may trigger diabetes in individuals with a diabetic ancestry and may cause a rise in blood fat in some susceptible individuals. The attempt by the sugar industry to differentiate between "quick-energy" and so-called "fattening" starches should deceive no one with a weight problem. And there has been no evidence to support the idea that eating sugar before meals cuts down the appetite and leads to significant weight reduction over a period of time. We certainly need additional evidence on the comparative roles of the various carbohydrates. On the basis of what we know, however, the replacement of a large part of the starch in the diet over the past centuries by sugar has not been favorable to health and has been disastrous to dental health.

Is it true that American bread is a terrible food, devitalized and almost useless?

This is an exaggerated statement. Lately, a great deal of food fanaticism seems to have focused on the subject of bread. Interest in the subject has been fanned by one or two sensational articles, by a controversy over advertising, and by a renewed

*See Appendix IV.

interest in the problem of vitamin and mineral enrichment. I believe that we have to look deeper, however, if we want to understand the passion with which bread is attacked.

Bread is still the staff of life, the Eucharist, the synonym for our daily sustenance. Yet everything we do not like about modern life, about industrialized society and technology, seems to be symbolized in modern bread.

Just look at the case presented against bread. White bread —by far the most common type sold and consumed in this country—is said to be a worthless food, contributing almost nothing to the diet except calories. It is true that present-day milling methods eliminate at least twenty nutrients, with only four or five put back into enriched bread. In addition, it appears that many people are dissatisfied with what they consider the insipidity of bread, which they associate with a lack of nutrition. Nevertheless, deficiencies and all, our enriched white bread is generally better than other countries' white breads.

Because I was born and raised in Paris, people speak to me with nostalgia for the Paris *boulangeries*, gleaming in marble and brass, with their great diversity of breads—from the long, thin baguette to the large, round loaf. The assumption is that these breads not only look highly decorative and smell and taste wonderful, but that they also represent a level of nutritional excellence way beyond the modern, soft, plastic-packaged American loaf.

As regards *nutrition*, our bread is better than the French bread and most other European breads. Professor Robert S. Harris of the Massachusetts Institute of Technology has studied the nutrient content of forty-four typical national breads, among them white enriched breads, including the U.S. standard loaf as well as nonenriched French, German, Italian and Swiss bread; enriched semiwhite wheat breads and nonenriched semiwhite breads; plus "wheat rye" and rye bread, mostly Scandinavian. The loaves were rated for their content of calcium, phosphorous, iron, thiamine, riboflavin, niacin, calcium pantothenate, vitamin B_6, protein, and the amino acids lysine, tryptophan, and methionine. Top rating went to a nonenriched semiwhite wheat bread from Finland. Second was the much-derided white enriched American bread, which had a good protein content (12 percent on a dry basis) and an excellent showing in all nutrients measured. French bread was *last* on a nutritional basis, with Italian, Swiss and German breads close competitors for the last place.

American bread makes a contribution to the diet, no matter how much some may want to believe it is as empty of nutrition as it is devoid of oomph. Indeed, at the end of World War II, two highly competent British nutritionists examined groups of German orphans who got over 70 percent of their daily calories from bread. The researchers could find no difference in health, growth and development between youngsters who ate whole-grain bread and those whose bread was white enriched. The rest of the diet was high in milk, meat and vegetables. Obviously, if the remainder of the diet had been sugar and fat, some differences might have emerged; but then it would have been a terrible diet anyway. In general, it is fair to say that whole-grain bread, "bran" bread and sprouted-wheat bread are better all around foods than white bread: they contribute some nutrients (B vitamins, vitamin E, and trace minerals) not found in white bread and they are also good sources of fiber. Absence of fiber in the diet has been correlated with development of diverticulitis and cancer of the large bowel, although the case is not yet proved.

Does bread have any other conspicuous merits?

It certainly does. Bread is our best card in our attempt to reduce fat in the diet. The Number One health problem (see Part II, Chapter Seven) in this country—both from the viewpoint of number of deaths and from that of number of people permanently disabled—is, overwhelmingly, heart disease. One factor in the veritable epidemic of cardiovascular diseases that has struck our country is high blood cholesterol, which in turn is related to the high-fat content of the diet. More fruits, more vegetables and more bread is the way we can modify the diet in order to lower the fat content.

Doesn't bread have a high overload of calories?

When it comes to the caloric content of bread, again we encounter misconceptions. Along with Johanna Dwyer, my **30** collaborator in the Nutrition Department at Harvard, I made a survey of people's beliefs about nutrition. We found that persons of all ages and walks of life (from high school students to physicians) tended grossly to overestimate the caloric content of bread. It is only about 60 calories a slice.

People *underestimate* the caloric content of meat (which runs to about 180 calories for a 3-ounce slice of roast beef; 340 calories for a 3-ounce hamburger or for a 3-ounce slice of ham).

You can, of course, load up a slice of bread with a lot of calories. If you put a restaurant-size pat of butter on your toast, for example, you triple the calories. Misconceptions about the calories in bread are actually a serious obstacle to the improvement of the American diet. Bread used to be—and should be again—an ideal carrier for nutrients that are low in the usual daily diet. Since American women often lack iron, the bakers have in fact petitioned the government for permission to double the iron-enrichment level. However, so long as teen-age girls and young women who need iron most go on believing that they only have to look at a piece of bread to put on twenty pounds, fortifying bread is not going to help much. Whole-wheat bread also contributes zinc and other trace minerals, as well as vitamin E. (These are also found, of course, in a variety of other foods.)

Are additives put into bread in many countries?

Throughout the world, additives are used in bread to give it qualities people find desirable. The most important have to do with the keeping qualities of bread. When I was a child in Paris, bread did not keep. It hardened rapidly and had to be bought fresh daily—or twice a day. Today French bread continues to look and taste like the bread of my childhood. It is made of bleached white flour because that is the way the French like it. It is unenriched because the French Academy of Medicine, rightly or wrongly, believes the variety of the French diet makes enrichment unnecessary. (Personally, I would have the flour enriched as insurance, but they make their own decisions.) But modern French women, like American women, do not want to be bothered with running twice daily to the bakeshop. And so additives are included which keep the bread from becoming

31   hard the same day it is baked and prevent the loaf from being visibly invaded by mold after two days. The practice is spreading throughout the world.

Isn't a great deal of whole-wheat bread consumed in this country?

Until recently, attempts by nutritionists to get people to eat whole-wheat bread have not been very successful. In spite of our efforts, people have gone on buying very little whole-wheat bread. And you can't blame the bread manufacturers for our low consumption of whole-wheat bread. They can easily shift the proportion of dark and white bread they make, and would do it if there were a demand. But the public taste has been slow to shift from what, for centuries, was the goal of every working family—to earn enough to be able to afford white bread every day.

Hasn't there been a change in the direction of dark bread in the past few years?

It may be that tastes are finally beginning to move that way. If so, this may be because so many of our young people have traveled to other parts of the world, or because there is a return to sophistication concerning the simple pleasures of life. Many people are now baking their own bread and derive great pleasure from developing an age-old skill. This is excellent. (Just be sure you don't spend 75 cents—or three hours—making a loaf that ends up being less nutritious than the humdrum store article. Use whole-grain or enriched flour and go easy on unnecessary high-caloric ingredients, such as butter, honey and molasses.)

Aren't there a greater number of choices available at the bread counters than there used to be?

More supermarkets and specialty stores are offering varieties of texture, shape and taste in bread. I'm leery of those heavy, darker breads that are overloaded with large amounts of shortening and molasses, needlessly doubling the caloric content of a sound article. But I am enthusiastic about many of the new varieties and with the idea that bread can be made interesting. The basic problem is still that people shun bread because they think it's fattening, and they think it's fattening because

32

it is so often totally unpalatable without butter on it. Bread that is good enough to eat unbuttered, or with just a small amount of butter or margarine, has few calories. This calls for imagination on the part of the breadmakers, and it's encouraging to see that efforts are already being made.

Our dentist is after us about sweets. Can the body really get along without them? Won't our diets be missing something?

For the answer, one has only to look at the many diabetics who get along without any sucrose at all. It is true that sucrose —table sugar—contains glucose as well as fructose (or fruit sugar). It is also true that the body burns glucose for energy. But the body is quite capable of making all the glucose it needs from more complex carbohydrates and, if necessary, from protein.

While some carbohydrate is essential to protect the body against the rise in blood ketones and the feeling of tiredness which accompanies diets excessively low in carbohydrates, the need for carbohydrates is just as well filled by starch, which usually accompanies otherwise valuable foods, most conspicuously bread and potatoes. And some nutritionists believe starch is far less harmful to teeth than is sugar. Sugar, whether spooned onto cereals, hidden in a hot dog, or taken as an unexpected part of a serving of corned beef hash, supplies nothing but empty calories. Of course, it is impractical to expect that sugar will disappear from the American diet. And there is nothing wrong with some sugar if you can afford it calorically after all your nutritional needs have been met—and if you brush or rinse your teeth after the meal. However, reducing the nation's sugar consumption would be a positive step toward coping with obesity, so often related to heart disease, and toward improving our dental health.

When the sugar ads claim that sugar is a source of "quick energy," does that mean that it is dissipated quickly and cannot be converted to fat?

Not on your life. Sugars can be converted into fat as easily as can other sources of calories. The "quick-energy" idea comes from the fact that it takes less time in your intestines for enzymes to split table sugar, a *di*saccharide (made from *two* simple sugars) than it takes to split starch which is a *poly*-saccharide (made from *hundreds* of simple sugar units linked together to make one giant molecule).

There are some good and some bad aspects to this quick rate of absorption.

The good news is that the quick absorption means that the glucose levels in blood go up fast. This phenomenon is probably related to the quick partial alleviation of hunger you get when you take a sugared drink or snack.

The bad news is that this quick rise in blood sugar stimulates a rapid increase in insulin, necessary for the utilization of sugar but also its deposition as fat. After this has occurred, insulin will cause a rapid drop in blood sugar with the reappearance of hunger in a more intense fashion.

How much sugar do we consume on the average in the U.S.? Do a few teaspoonfuls a day really add up to a nutrition problem?

Our consumption is high: 105 pounds per person per year (or 500 calories a day). We also consume about 15 pounds of corn syrup per year. And while our total food consumption is going down, our sugar consumption has stayed steady. Our annual consumption of sugar is roughly the equivalent, in terms of body fat, of about 50 pounds. So it's obvious that sugar, as a source of "empty calories" (calories unaccompanied by any nutrients), is one of the first foods to cut down on (or cut out altogether) when on a reducing diet. Sugar consumption is, unfortunately, not just in the "a few teaspoonsful a day" category. It has become almost all-pervasive. Its presence is clear in candy, cake, cookies, pies and the syrups in canned and frozen fruit. It is also in beans, soups, cereals, baby vegetables, canned ham and a myriad of other products. (Go around your kitchen and check the labels.)

But has sugar not always been one of our major sources of calories?

The Greeks and Romans knew nothing of table sugar. It is not mentioned in the Bible, the Talmud or the Koran. It was not until the end of the fifteenth century that consignments of cane sugar arrived in Europe. And the massive consumption of sugar observed in present-day Western countries is new. For example, we have good data for England, where almost all sugar is imported and goes through customs. In 1830 the average consumption of sugar in England was on the order of 5 pounds per person per year. Now it is 125 pounds. Cane and beet sugar consumption in the United States went from nothing at the time of the Pilgrims to 105 pounds per person now!

Is there much difference nutritionally between white and brown sugars?

Not enough to matter. White sugar offers nothing except calories. Brown sugar contains traces of nutrients, but in amounts so small as to be insignificant. Molasses, on the other hand, still retains nutrients, such as iron, calcium and some of the B vitamins, but in variable and unreliable amounts.

Please comment on the nutritional value of honey.

Although the lore on honey hunting, beekeeping, and the use of honey in myth and religious ritual is fascinating, the reputation of honey as a medicinal or nutritious food is undeserved. Honey contains about 75 percent sugar and 20 percent water and holds approximately 65 calories per tablespoon. Despite claims of superior nutritional benefits by honey-lovers, the fact is that honey, like other sugars, is virtually devoid of other nutrients. Honey was the major sweetener available in the Western world until fairly late in history when sucrose was introduced through trade with the Indies. At first it was used only in making medicines. It was not until after the fifteenth century that sucrose production increased to the point where it began to replace honey as a sweetener.

Honey consumption has become increasingly popular in recent years, particularly as a result of the interest in so-called natural foods. There are almost endless varieties of nectars to choose from, each with a characteristic flavor. Even with this increased use of honey, the average annual per capita consumption in the United States is not much more than two pounds compared to over a hundred pounds of sugar. While there is no reason to recommend an increased consumption of honey, it is imperative, as I have said many times before, that we decrease our sugar consumption. It is preferable to get your carbohydrates from fruits, vegetables and potatoes and whole-grain cereals. This way, they act as carriers for a multitude of useful nutrients.

Could you please evaluate the nutrient content of refined sugar, "raw" sugar, maple syrup, and corn syrup?

In two simple words: hardly any. What you're really talking about is just a difference in sources. The calories, per tablespoon, do vary a little, from 45 for white sugar to 60 for corn syrup, a highly concentrated solution.

"Raw" sugar, as it is sold in the United States, is in reality ordinary sucrose or table sugar with cane fiber or beet pulp added to give it the approximate texture and taste of real raw sugar, which contains too many impurities to pass federal inspection.

What is the status of saccharin? Is it safe to use as much as I want?

The Food and Drug Administration currently recommends restricting one's intake of saccharin to no more than 1 gram a day. In terms of every-day foods this amounts to seven 12-ounce bottles of diet soda or sixty small saccharin tablets a day—considerably more than anyone is probably taking. Once in a while there is a saccharin "scare"—new work which according to some suggests that taking saccharin is dangerous. So far, this work has not convinced the Food and Drug Administration—nor the Committee of the National Academy of Sciences consulted by FDA on the possible toxicity of saccharin.

The FDA has set limits on the amounts which can be added in the manufacture of diet foods. The amount a product contains must clearly be stated on the label, so you will be able to calculate your own daily saccharin intake.

The FDA actions followed a preliminary report that bladder tumors were discovered in animals fed massive doses of the sweetener. Actually the animals were given an amount that is equivalent to 875 bottles of diet soda per day. If the tumors are verified, and if they are not produced solely as the result of the high concentration in the experiments (that is, crystals of saccharin acting as an irritant), the government will have to invoke the so-called Delaney clause and saccharin will probably be banned.

Meanwhile, the FDA and a committee of the National Research Council–National Academy of Sciences are watching the situation carefully. I would personally hesitate to recommend saccharin because of the remaining doubts about its safety, but I can tell you that I use it in my tea or coffee. On the other hand, I am careful to interrupt my use of it for a day or two every four or five days to prevent its accumulating. If you have a sweet tooth (and are not diabetic, and don't have fragile teeth) the answer is still sugar—considerably reduced in amount.

Can you describe the potential of the artichoke as a sugar substitute?

As far back as 1935 it was noted in scientific literature that certain beverages taste sweet after one has eaten artichokes. French cookbooks, in fact, often advise against wine with artichokes because it will taste undesirably sweet.

New investigation of the artichoke as a potential nonnutritive sweetener is related to the taste-bud approach to changing food flavors. Tests have shown that one-fourth of an artichoke heart on the tongue tastes twice as sweet as two teaspoons of sugar in six ounces of water. The effect lasts four or five minutes. Interestingly, thirty-four of the forty subjects involved in the test noted this effect; all six who did not were males. Two chemicals, cynarin and chlorogenic acid, isolated from artichokes, are believed to be largely, though not totally, responsible for its sweetening ability. (A more interesting, "natural" sweetener is "miracle fruit," an African berry which contains a protein that activates taste buds for about one hour, making sour or slightly sweet foods quite sweet—and unsalted meats satisfactorily salty.)

5
VITAMINS- THE MORE, THE MURKIER

The body is a versatile chemist. It makes thousands of different substances. There are, however, some things it cannot produce: some of the fatty acids and some of the amino acids. We call these necessary fatty acids and amino acids the "essential fatty acids" (or polyunsaturates) and the "essential amino acids." There are some other complex substances the body needs in small amounts and that it is unable to manufacture. These are called the vitamins. They must be provided by foods (or by "vitamin supplements") or the body will not function at peak efficiency. A serious shortage of one or more vitamins will cause one or more deficiency diseases; extreme deficiencies are fatal.*

Most vitamins are designated by a letter of the alphabet because at one time we did not know their chemical structure and could not give them a proper scientific name. In addition, there are vitamins which have proved to be two or more related substances with similar roles in the body. For example, there are several "vitamins D." In some cases, a substance found in food is a "provitamin" which, when consumed, is transformed into the needed vitamin itself. For instance, there are various carotenes which, after being eaten, become vitamin A.

*See Appendix V.

The vitamins are usually divided into "water-soluble vitamins," found in the watery parts of cells (and foods), and the "fat-soluble vitamins" which are dissolved in fat or in the fat part of cells. The fat-soluble vitamins are A, D, E and K. The water-soluble vitamins are vitamin B, in particular B_1, B_2, niacin, pyridoxine, B_{12}, folic acid, biotin, and pantothenic acid, and vitamin C.

Vitamin A is found in nature as the provitamin, carotene, in green and yellow plants and as two forms of the vitamin itself in fresh-water fish and land animals, on the one hand, and sea fish and animals, on the other. It is also found in summer butter, which is butter churned from milk collected in the summer when the cows eat fresh grass full of carotene, the splitting of which in the organism gives rise to vitamin A. Vitamin A then goes on to be secreted in the milk. (In "Golden Guernseys" the splitting is incomplete; some of the yellow carotene pigment is secreted into the milk unchanged—hence the golden color of the milk.) Vitamin A is essential in the growth and maintenance of epithelial tissue which comprises the skin and the covering of internal cavities. It is important in the harmonious development of the bones. It is a constituent in the maintenance of the outside of the eye and is also made into a pigment in the retina of the eye which enables us to see. This pigment is involved in a complex photochemical process essential to night and twilight vision.

Vitamin D is found in certain foods (fish liver oil, liver, eggs, summer butter) and is also formed when the skin is exposed to the sun. Because cows are exposed to sunshine in pastures, they manufacture vitamin D by conversion of cholesterol. Some of the vitamin D then is secreted into the milk and, being like vitamin A fat-soluble, ends up in the butter fraction. Vitamin D is necessary for the utilization of the mineral calcium. Milk is often fortified with vitamin D to the level of 400 I.U. (the Recommended Dietary Allowance) per quart.

Vitamin E has a number of important roles which have been described in animals. So far, vitamin E deficiency has not been identified clearly in man, except perhaps in situations where fat absorption is grievously impaired.

Vitamin K, indispensable for the proper clotting of blood, is normally manufactured by bacteria in the intestine. Newborn babies who do not yet have bacteria in their intestines often need a supplement of vitamin K.

Vitamin B_1 (also called thiamine) is found in whole-grain cereals and meat, among other sources. It is needed for the utilization of starches and sugars.

Vitamin B_2 also is essential to a number of chemical reactions whereby food is utilized in the body.

Niacin (nicotinic acid and nicotinic acid amide, also called vitamin P or PP) is necessary for the respiration of the cells. The amino acid tryptophan can be changed into niacin in the body.

Pyridoxine is a vitamin involved in many chemical reactions, in particular in the utilization of protein.

Pantothenic acid and biotin are also known to be necessary factors.

Folic acid and vitamin B_{12} are needed for the formation of red cells. B_{12} is also necessary for the maintenance of certain nerves.

Vitamin C, ascorbic acid, found in fruit (in particular in oranges and lemons) and potatoes, is necessary for the maintenance of connective tissue, the tissue that binds together the various organs.

What are the results of not getting enough vitamins?

Vitamin A deficiency causes night blindness, lack of vision in dim light, and blinding by sudden exposure to light. It also causes abnormalities of the mucosa and dry, itchy skin. Blindness and death result from extreme deficiency of this vitamin.

Vitamin B_1 deficiency, known also as beriberi, is widespread in Asia and elsewhere particularly where polished rice is the main food. It causes nerve damage, a type of heart disease, and edema (swelling). Vitamin B_2 deficiency causes cracking at the corners of the lips and itching.

The deficiency disease pellagra, characterized by skin disease, diarrhea and insanity (the three D's: Dermatitis, Diarrhea and Dementia—with eventually Death occurring), is found when the diet is low in protein (generally animal protein) containing the amino acid tryptophan as well as low in niacin, another B vitamin.

In the United States, flour is enriched with vitamins B_1 and B_2, niacin and iron. Corn is low in niacin and tryptophan, and persons in the South who eat mostly corn with little or no animal protein used to develop pellagra. Corn is now enriched in the United States, and the number of persons with pellagra has been radically reduced.

Lack of pyridoxine (vitamin B_6) causes convulsions in infants.

Lack of folic acid (a B vitamin) and of vitamin B_{12} causes blood disorders in which abnormal red cells are formed. The nervous system is affected when B_{12} is lacking.

Vitamin C deficiency, more familiarly known as scurvy, the scourge for centuries of seafarers and others who were deprived of fresh fruits for long periods, makes joints painful, causes sore and bleeding gums and makes wounds slow to heal. It also weakens the walls of the capillaries (very small blood vessels), causing them to break easily.

Vitamin D deficiency prevents calcium from being properly deposited in the bones, and in young children causes such abnormal development of the bones as knock-knees and "pigeon breast." This condition is known also as rickets. Adult rickets, known as osteomalacia, is a similar softening and deformation of the bones.

If 10 milligrams of a particular vitamin are good for you, does it not follow that 500 milligrams of it will be 50 times better?

No, not at all. In fact, enormous amounts can be harmful! Let me explain. From California to the Atlantic Coast (the usual route for diet fads is from west to east, like the prevailing winds), an unbelievable quantity of people are taking enormous amounts of one particular vitamin after the other in dosages a hundred or even thousands of times greater than the amount needed to prevent dietary deficiency.

Vitamin C was the first of these recent megavitamin fads. Vitamin E is now the up-and-coming passion, and it's not hard to foresee that the whole alphabet of vitamins will soon be worked through.

How did the vitamin C craze get started?

It was launched through the totally honest and disinterested enthusiasm of Professor Linus Pauling. He is among the greatest of contemporary chemists. His discoveries of the structure of a number of extremely complicated organic molecules, such as the abnormal hemoglobin in the blood of persons with sickle cell anemia, were properly rewarded by the Nobel Prize in Chemistry. His notable efforts to call attention to the genetic damage caused by atmospheric atomic explosions were instrumental in bringing about an international ban which has been respected by three of the five atomic powers. This great achievement was acknowledged by the award to Dr. Pauling of the Nobel Prize for Peace.

None of this invalidates Will Rogers' wise maxim that "We are all ignorant about different things." In Professor Pauling's case, the weak spot seems to be epidemiology, the difficult discipline that deals with the evaluation of medical statistics about people—a far cry from organic chemistry.

Did the conclusions of epidemiologists differ from those of Linus Pauling?

They did. Looking at the same facts, the epidemiologists could see no definitive evidence that gigantic doses of vitamin C had a substantial effect in curing or preventing the common cold. Later data, collected from a careful experiment in a large prison, also failed to document ascorbic acid (vitamin C) as a cure or preventive for that most prevalent of all human ills. Some recent data, in particular those obtained in Canada in military populations, do suggest a slight effect in preventing or cutting down on the length of the common cold. Other studies do not find *any* effects. Even in the "positive" studies, the effect is far from impressive. Yet, some of our fellow Americans are taking 500 milligrams, 1,000 milligrams, or even more of the vitamin every day. The minimum dose needed—to prevent scurvy, which is what vitamin C is mostly all about—is some 10 mg. per day. The recommended daily intake, aiming to provide a large margin of safety, has been set at 30 mg. per day by international organizations and by the British Medical Council. For extra assurance, the Food and Nutrition Board of the U.S. National Research Council–National Academy of Sciences recommends 45 to 60 mg. daily (we are richer). I had occasion not long ago to speak to a man who was taking 30 grams daily. That's 3,000 times the antiscorbutic (antiscurvy) dose!

What particular danger is involved in these giant doses of vitamin C?

We have absolutely no data on the long-run safety of doses of this magnitude. Moderate excesses—such as 100 mg. per day —are excreted in the urine without any side effect. Enormous doses produce an acidic urine which sometimes causes burning sensations. These disappear when the vitamin C intake is brought down to reasonable levels. Very acidic urine may also cause the formation and movement of "gravel" in persons prone to urinary stones. One recent study suggests the possibility that large doses of vitamin C may destroy substantial amounts of the vitamin B_{12} in foods during digestion in the intestinal tract.

As far as what goes on in tissues and organs, it can't be emphasized enough that we *just do not know* what this supersaturation with ascorbic acid does. I find it remarkable that some of the people who are most nervous about what they call "untested chemicals in our food" nevertheless dose themselves daily with a substance that is needed (and well understood) at the required levels but is actually an "untested chemical" when taken in huge doses.

What is actually known about vitamin E and our need for it?

Vitamin E is really a group of four closely related compounds. It is certainly needed by man, though its role in health is not well understood. Vitamin E deficiency causes tissue swelling and brain damage in chickens and faulty development of the placenta and destruction of the fetus in female rats, mice, hamsters and guinea pigs. It produces testicular degeneration in male rodents of several species, a kind of muscular dystrophy (different from the human disease) in rabbits, degeneration of the heart muscle and heart failure in calves, anemia in monkeys,

43

and fragility with easy damage of the red blood cells in rats *and* men.

Because of the variety of the deficiency signs in various animals, enormous doses of vitamin E have been tried in a great many human diseases, from habitual abortion to heart disease and muscular dystrophy. The experiments were not a success. So doctors went back to the position that we need vitamin E, but only in moderate amounts.

Are there times when we need more vitamin E than the recommended daily allowance?

We do need more of it when we eat more polyunsaturated fats in order to lower cholesterol. This is because vitamin E acts as an antioxidant—a substance which protects other molecules from combining with oxygen to form toxic "peroxides." But enormous amounts seem to confer no special benefit. The requirement had been set at 30 international units a day. It has recently been lowered to 15 units a day by the Food and Nutrition Board of the National Academy of Sciences–National Research Council. You can easily get that much if you eat plenty of fruits, vegetables, and whole-grains and corn, soybean, peanut, or cottonseed oil. Yet thousands of people are taking 400 international units or more a day. The rationale seems to come from recent experiments suggesting that mice given large amounts of *other* ("synthetic") antioxidants—not vitamin E—lived longer than expected. Even though too many Americans are on diets that are probably too low in vitamin E, this isn't sufficient reason to jump into the *terra incognita* of overdosage.

Can you name some vitamins that could be likely candidates for promotion of fads?

Vitamin B_1 deficiency in people causes loss of appetite, fatigue, irritability, neuritis and headaches. But there is no evidence that more than the basic daily requirement of 1 to 1.5 mg. will do any good when these signs and symptoms are due to other causes, which they often are.

Vitamin B_{12}, the "growth" or "miracle" or "red" vitamin, was the last major vitamin to be discovered. Because people who were deficient in this vitamin didn't grow at a normal rate, there were early hopes it could help slow growers grow faster —even if they weren't vitamin B_{12} deficient. It didn't. However, with its galaxy of nicknames, how could it fail to find a market? Many patients still insist upon asking for vitamin B_{12} "shots" when they feel run down.

Vitamin D is and has always been "the sunshine vitamin," so-called because a deficiency of D causes rickets, which can also be cured by sufficient exposure to sunshine. All children need a supplement of vitamin D (in pills or in vitamin D–enriched milk) at the level of 400 international units a day. At various times it has been falsely claimed that vitamin D in very large doses is useful in a whole range of non-nutritional diseases, from arthritis and asthma to schizophrenia and tuberculosis. Not only have these claims not been confirmed, but it has become clear that daily doses much in excess of the Recommended Dietary Allowance of 400 international units are dangerous. The Food and Drug Administration would probably move very quickly against any promotion of very large doses and is, in fact, attempting to have large doses of vitamin D classified as prescription drugs. They are also attempting to put large doses of vitamin A in the same category. Too many adolescents are convinced that massive doses of vitamin A will cure or prevent acne, a hope which, unfortunately, is not based on any evidence.

Surrounded as we are by the elaborate claims for vitamins in monster doses and with prospects of more to come, what is the soundest position for a layman to take?

Remember that you need vitamins, all vitamins, each day —not C last year and E this year and X or Y or Z next year. The daily allowances recommended by the National Research Council are established by subcommittees of the best experts on each vitamin.* These are men and women with research experience with these vitamins in clinical nutrition.

The allowances contain a generous but reasonable margin of safety to cover individual differences and changing conditions. Large doses much in excess of the allowances are needed only in certain disease states and should be taken only by prescription of a physician.

A varied diet with plenty of fruits and vegetables, fortified

*See Appendix VI.

milk, and a reasonable amount of animal products (not excessive in fat) and very little sugar, soft drinks or alcohol provides the nutrients you need.

If your physician advises it, a supplement of one vitamin pill containing *no more than* the recommended daily allowances of all required vitamins and iron can be taken, particularly if your food habits are irregular or if you are on a strenuous reducing diet. As far as the megavitamins are concerned, remember this: in normal amounts, vitamins are food; at five, ten, a hundred, or a thousand times the normal level, vitamins are drugs and should be treated accordingly.

Promotional pieces speak of "natural" as opposed to "synthetic" vitamins, claiming or implying superiority of the former over the latter. Are there differences?

"Natural" vitamins, to go along with an unnecessary and meaningless distinction, are those that are in food or produced in the body by provitamins in food. "Synthetic" vitamins are those produced in a factory. Incidentally, they were brought into being by people called "organic" chemists. Natural vitamins are no better than synthetic vitamins. They have exactly the same atoms in their molecules, arranged in exactly the same way. They're the same things in their chemical behavior. A vitamin is a vitamin is a vitamin. Oh, yes. Frequently the so-called natural vitamins—let's stop being polite!—cost more money.

The other day I was eating a doughnut and, to my surprise, I read on the box that it was vitamin enriched. I found that the vitamin values given were for three ounces of doughnut. A little arithmetic revealed that this meant two doughnuts, not one. Anyway, it seemed to me that even two doughnuts didn't contain much nutrition. How do they stack up against a slice of bread, for example?

In comparing a store brand of enriched doughnuts with a store brand of sliced white bread (the latter costing in late 1974 about 2 cents and the former costing about 8 cents), each contains almost the same amount of thiamine, riboflavin, niacin and iron. But the slice of bread contains about 60 calories and the doughnut more than three times as many, or 185.

The obvious conclusion: although it is good that some doughnuts are being made with enriched flour and provide something more than empty calories, the role of doughnuts as something more than an occasional treat in the market basket must be seriously questioned because of their cost and high calories.

Is it all right to keep frozen orange juice for a couple of days after it is made? I've heard that it quickly loses all of its vitamin C. Is this true?

Orange juice frozen by modern commercial methods should be equal in ascorbic acid to the freshly squeezed product. If the oranges used to make the fresh juice were quite underripe when picked and then sat around for some time at room temperature, the frozen variety may be better.

It is true that ascorbic acid is a highly perishable vitamin. In order to keep your orange juice at its nutritional best, it should be stored in a glass or plastic (not metal) covered container and kept cool. By following these procedures, you can certainly keep orange juice for a few days without fear of significant nutrient loss.

Are cooked carrots better for you than raw ones?

Yes and no. Raw carrots are among the few foods that have any texture to them that both children and adults will eat. This is fine for your teeth and gums. They are also a good source of fiber (roughage). On the other hand, the carotene (which turns into vitamin A) is more available if the carrots are softened by cooking. My advice: eat them both ways.

I gather that you are not very enthusiastic for wheat-germ oil and (killed) brewer's yeast. Yet these are good sources of vitamin E and the B vitamins, respectively. What accounts for your attitude?

The items you mention are good dietary supplements. But if you have an otherwise well-balanced diet with plenty of fruits and vegetables and with whole-grain and animal products, you should not need dietary supplements. If your physician feels you need a supplement as "insurance," he or she will prescribe **47** a complete vitamin-mineral combination, not above the levels of the Recommended Dietary Allowance, made by a reputable manufacturer. Infants and children, not exposed to sunshine in winter months, require vitamin D, either in milk or in a vitamin supplement.

> *I am sixty-five years old. A friend of about the same age is getting vitamin B_{12} shots to give her more energy. She claims to feel better. Are B_{12} injections a good idea for those of us who feel more sluggish than we like?*

No. Vitamin B_{12} is among the nutrients which have too often been given in massive doses needlessly and without scientific reason. The only indication for injections of B_{12} is for a specific condition—pernicious anemia, where the individual cannot properly use the B_{12} he or she consumes.

Vitamin B_{12}, essential to the functioning of all body cells, is widely available in foods of animal origin. A deficiency, as a result of dietary intake, has been observed in people eating only vegetables. Although scientific evidence shows that the ability to use B_{12} does decrease with age, a well-balanced diet should still provide you with all you need.

> *If you eat for breakfast a bowl of cereal that contains 100 percent of your daily requirement of vitamins, is it all right to eat anything you like the rest of the day?*

Those added vitamins are usually only some of the major ones for which a Recommended Daily Allowance has been established. You need a great many other nutrients, such as those minerals that are essential to life. For example, the body needs phosphorous, calcium and magnesium for strong teeth and bones, zinc for growth, chromium for the utilization of carbohydrates, and copper for hemoglobin, to mention only a few. You certainly still need a good diet the rest of the day.

> *I have heard that schizophrenia could be improved or cured through the use of massive quantities ("megadoses") of certain vitamins, particularly niacin. Any truth to this?*

None. The American Psychiatric Association had a highly qualified task force examine fourteen controlled studies on the use of megadoses of niacin in schizophrenia. The conclusion of the report: niacin was of no use in the treatment of this disease.

6 MINERALS—MAJOR AND MINI

One may not think of food as something to be mined in addition to being planted, bred and hunted or fished for. But many of man's most important nutrients are scratched from the crust of the earth. Several of these minerals, needed by the body in relatively large amounts, are: calcium, phosphorous, magnesium, iron, sodium, potassium, sulfur and chlorine.

Throughout our lives we need fresh supplies of calcium to replace that which is constantly called upon to perform necessary functions. Ninety-nine percent of our calcium is in our skeleton, all but 1 percent of which is in the bones, the rest in the teeth. The remaining 1 percent which is not in the skeleton makes the muscles, including the heart, contract; aids in blood clotting; and is concerned with the nourishment of cells, the conversion of food to energy, and the supply of an ingredient that facilitates the transmission of nerve impulses.*

The Recommended Daily Allowance of calcium for ordinary adults is set at 800 milligrams (equivalent to the calcium in about two glasses of milk) a day. Requirements are higher for other groups: equivalent to three glasses of milk a day for

*See Appendix V.

children and pregnant women, four for adolescents, and at least four for nursing mothers. Yogurt, hard cheeses and small fish (eaten bones and all) are excellent sources for those who dislike milk or are unable to tolerate it. Softer cheeses, dark green leafy vegetables, broccoli, baked beans, dried figs and dried legumes are also good calcium sources.

Closely allied in the body with calcium and vitamin D is phosphorous. It is mostly in the skeleton and accounts for about 1 percent of body weight. Phosphorous is also essential for the chemical reactions whereby energy is transferred from food for the synthesis of body substances and for changing chemical into electrical energy in the nerves and muscles. We get phosphorous from milk and lean meats, fish and vegetables. The daily requirement is the same as for calcium: 800 mg. per day.

There is about one ounce of magnesium in the body of an adult. Much of it is combined with calcium and phosphorous in the bone. The remainder is in red blood cells and in body fluids. We need magnesium to keep hormones working, to use carbohydrates for energy and to maintain muscles.

The requirement for magnesium has been set for women at 300, and for men at 350 milligrams a day; for infants and children from 60 to 250 a day; and for pregnant and nursing women, 450. Rats and monkeys fed diets extremely low in magnesium showed much more extensive cholesterol deposits and hardening of arteries when fed diets containing large amounts of cholesterol. There is no reason to suppose, however, that magnesium supplements will in any way prevent the development of atherosclerosis in an individual on a satisfactory diet. And, indeed, there are many sources of magnesium: large amounts in whole-grain cereals (especially oats), milk, fish and shellfish (particularly shrimp), and in meat, fruit, vegetables and nuts.

Iron is an essential part of hemoglobin, the pigment of red blood cells which loosely combines in the lungs with oxygen and carries it to all the tissues. The most common anemia seen in this country is iron-deficiency anemia. It is seen in infants and young children and in women of childbearing age. Dr. Stanley Gershoff of our Nutrition Department at Harvard has found it to be more common among the elderly of both sexes than had been suspected.

For infants, iron requirements (10–15 mg. per day) can easily be met by continuing to use baby cereals as long as the child will accept them. Meeting the iron needs of older children and women through diet is a much greater problem. Their requirement has been set at 18 mg. per day. Many experts feel that meeting it is, in fact, impossible, and that many women should take iron supplements. There is, however, merit in attempting to include as much iron as possible in the diet.

Liver and kidney are the best iron sources. Others include oysters, shrimp, sardines, most meats, dried beans, most nuts, eggs, prunes, raisins, green leafy vegetables and enriched bread and cereals. The level of iron in enriched bread may be increased soon.

The elderly pose a difficult problem, because often their overall intake of food is very low. Again, the idea is to increase the iron concentration in the diet by serving the foods I have just mentioned and to resort to iron supplements only if absolutely necessary.

Sodium is found mainly in the blood, lymph and digestive juices and the fluid which bathes cells. About a fifth of one percent of the body is sodium, a third of which is in the skeleton. The average American seems to eat about ten times as much sodium chloride (table salt) as he requires. Most people would do well to banish the salt shaker from the dining room table. They could satisfy their needs for sodium from reasonable amounts of milk, meat, eggs, carrots, beets and spinach. For people with a family history of hypertension, cutting down on salt is extremely prudent.

Chlorine exists throughout the body and particularly in the acid in the stomach which digests food. You can meet all your requirement for chlorine from the slightest amount of table salt.

Sulfur used by the body comes from two amino acids (cystine and methionine) each of which contains sulfur. It is an ingredient of hair, nails, bones, tendons and the fluids of our joints. It performs a function in the process by which the body rids itself of common poisonous substances. It is provided by lean meat, fish, fruits and vegetables.

The body has about twice as much potassium as sodium and most of it is within the cells. Potassium is vital for maintaining the chemical balance of the cellular fluids. A small additional amount is required for the work of the muscles, especially the heart muscle. There is plenty of potassium in oranges, bananas, dried fruits, tomatoes, leafy vegetables, peas and beans, meats and fish.

People who lose sodium when they take drugs to lower their blood pressure also lose potassium and thus need more in their diet or in special supplements.

Here are some typical questions I am asked on this aspect of nutrition.

I've been told that rhubarb, spinach and beet greens work against the absorption of calcium. Is this true? And, if true, can anything be done about it?

Yes and yes. Rhubarb, spinach, chard, beet greens and whole grains do work against the proper absorption of dietary calcium. Anyone who ate only these foods would be well on the way to a calcium-deficiency problem. But most people scatter these foods among scores of other choices. Thus the amount of calcium that fails to be absorbed will be small and the occasions when it will happen will be infrequent. Another bow for the varied diet.

Does cow's milk supply more calcium than mother's milk?

Cow's milk indeed supplies more of certain nutrients, including calcium, than mother's milk. Whether this represents an advantage or a disadvantage when the cow's milk is fed to very young infants, we don't know. I endorse well-known Philadelphia pediatrician and nutritionist Dr. Paul Gyorgy's statement that "mother's milk is for infants, cow's milk is for calves."

I always take what I'm told is a sufficient amount of calcium a day, but I don't seem to be getting any benefit from it. A neighbor suggests that I take vitamin-D capsules. Do you agree?

You may be getting plenty of calcium in your diet, but not getting full value of it because you're missing some of the other nutrients required to help the body use calcium. Vitamin D is, of course, essential. You can get it easily in vitamin D–enriched milk. In the summer, you can get it from sufficient daily exposure to sunshine. Small children in northern climates should receive a vitamin D supplement if their milk is not fortified. Nonpregnant, non-nursing adults usually do well without a supplement if they eat a varied diet.

My children do not care for liver or for spinach. How can they get the iron they need?

If they don't like liver, that is unfortunate. You should work harder to get them to eat it. Use your imagination and your cookbooks. There are many attractive ways to cook liver. And don't forget chicken livers, which are just as nutritious as beef or calf. And which children often like. As for spinach, many children don't eat it because their mothers make faces over it and their fathers make jokes about it. If the children persist in refusing to eat liver and spinach, don't worry about it. Try other sources of iron such as dried apricots or figs.

There are so many good recipes that require salt. Why can't potassium chloride be used as a substitute for people on a salt-free diet?

Potassium chloride, as well as other potassium salts, can be used as a sodium chloride substitute. But, since some individuals cannot tolerate increased amounts of potassium, these products should be used only with the doctor's consent. Unfortunately, salt substitutes don't taste much like regular salt, and individuals must develop a taste for them. Moreover, you just can't replace a heavy hand on the salt shaker with a heavy hand on the salt-substitute shaker.

In general, a more successful practice is for people on sodium-restricted diets to use herbs and spices more effectively in cooking. Mustard, cinnamon, nutmeg, garlic, oregano, thyme, chives, dill and lemon can be used in almost any amounts. But remember: "seasoned" salts such as garlic salt, onion salt, and celery salt all contain regular salt and should be avoided if you're on a salt-free diet.

I'd always thought that I was eating a well-balanced diet with plenty of foods high in calcium. I was upset to find that I have osteoporosis. Isn't that a calcium deficiency? Is there any dietary treatment?

Osteoporosis is a general decrease in the bone minerals and eventually the bone mass of the body. With few exceptions, it is a phenomenon of the aging process. The demineralization begins at around age forty and continues from then on. There is an increased incidence of osteoporosis with aging. It has been said that in anyone who lives long enough its development is inevitable.

The cause remains elusive. It occurs far more frequently in women than in men, a factor attributed to post-menopausal hormonal changes. Other factors thought to contribute to its development include insufficient physical activity. In one large study, a greater incidence of osteoporosis was observed in low-fluoride areas than in a community where the water supply naturally contained large amounts of fluoride.

Just as the cause remains a mystery, satisfactory treatment has not as yet been found. Unfortunately, large doses of calcium do not result in a remineralization of bone. Recently, it has been suggested that a decrease in the acidity of the "ash," or residue, of the diet might be effective in slowing the rate of calcium loss from bone. In men who generally eat an omnivorous diet, the residue is acid; in vegetarians it is alkaline. It has been suggested that in omnivorous men calcium loss is hastened. In one study, x-ray showed a greater decrease in bone density among meat-eaters than among vegetarians. The idea of using a diet to promote the formation of an alkaline ash, including lots of fruits, vegetables, vegetable proteins with limited milk and less meat, is interesting and deserves further investigation.

Prevention is obviously the ultimate goal. Meanwhile, increased physical activity and a diet adequate in calcium and vitamin D are certainly appropriate measures.

Not long ago you disputed the idea, presented by a popular writer on nutrition, that magnesium is "nature's tranquilizer." Reading the same book, I was interested in her claim that a social drinker who takes a daily cocktail containing two ounces of alcohol excretes from three to five times as much magnesium as is normal. She maintained that if that drinker doesn't take a daily magnesium supplement "he's asking for a heart attack." What is the relationship between magnesium, alcohol and heart attacks?

I believe that probably she had put together a set of independent findings and drawn a conclusion that research in the field simply cannot support. Let's examine the facts.

It is true that some chronic alcoholics have low levels of magnesium in their blood and that after alcohol ingestion excretion of magnesium may be increased. It is true also that in laboratory studies rats and monkeys given atherogenic diets, also low in magnesium, are more susceptible to atherosclerosis. While it is obviously important to study the relationship between magnesium and atherosclerosis in man, I think you can agree that, on the basis of the facts currently available, it seems a bit premature to recommend that a Scotch and soda before dinner include a dash of magnesium carbonate.

Some time ago, my mother told me to stop using iron cookware because it contained traces of copper. She said that copper destroys vitamins and possibly is poisonous. Is this true?

Both copper and iron do destroy vitamin C. For this reason, a food like cabbage, which is high in vitamin C, should be steamed in an aluminum or stainless steel pot.

But that is only part of the story. Copper is, in fact, an essential nutrient for man, although only minute amounts are needed. It's necessary for the formation and development of red blood cells and is found in a number of enzymes as well. Excessive amounts of copper may be toxic, but certainly not the negligible amounts obtained from eating food cooked even in all-copper pots.

Cooking in iron pots is quite safe, even if they happen to contain traces of copper. Since iron dissolves during the cooking process, foods cooked in iron pots can also contribute substantially to the day's iron requirements.

And now, for a few words about the mini-minerals, from aluminum to zinc.

People have used iodized salt for so long that probably half of us have forgotten why salt is iodized. In fact, iodization was the first, most dramatic, example of a practice that is now commonplace: the wholesale addition of a vital nutrient to an everyday food to satisfy a need unfilled by the usual diet.

Iodine is what we call a trace mineral. And people who don't get a natural supply of it—by eating seafood, for example—may be afflicted with goiter. This is one of the most clear-cut cases of what can happen when people are deficient in even the tiniest, almost-impossible-to-measure quantities of these essential trace elements or trace minerals. Our need for iodine is measured in micrograms—130 per day for men, 100 for women.

Iodine is an essential component of the thyroid-gland hormones that regulate the rate at which our tissues breathe. Without it, the tissues use less oxygen, the body slows down, and eventually so does the mind. The thyroid gland enlarges in an attempt to compensate for the lack of iodine, causing the typical swelling of the neck we know as simple goiter. Goiter practically disappeared from the United States when table salt was iodized and people living in parts of the country where the soil had little or no iodine began eating food from other sections.

Lately, however, the use of iodized salt has dwindled and goiter has reappeared in iodine-deficient areas where impoverished people have a monotonous and poorly balanced diet.

About one half the iodine in the human body is in the muscles. About a fifth is in the thyroid, the rest in the skin, the skeleton and other tissues. Its important role in the thyroid is to take part in the synthesis of the thyroid hormones which control the rate at which the principal chemical reactions of the body occur. The rest of the trace-mineral story is less simple. Not even the nutrition experts know *all* they would like to know about trace minerals—how they work, why the body needs them, what foods are rich in them, or even whether we know them all. And our lack of knowledge creates a fertile field for propaganda, confusion and fear.

Is it true that, as "health-food" purveyors insist, the use of chemical fertilizers "devitalizes" our foods by depriving them of trace minerals?

There is no evidence that this is so. First, if the soil is in fact deficient in one or several key trace minerals, the plants do not grow. They require most trace minerals as we (and farm animals) also do. There are minerals which they do not seem to need—such as fluoride or iodine—but then, if these are absent from the soil or the water, farm animals also lack them, and the manure from these animals lacks them too. Fertilizers used in deficient soil do in fact include trace minerals missing in these areas—otherwise we would get no crop.

Does this mean that we don't have to worry about trace minerals in the diet?

I did not say that. If we attempt to subsist entirely on highly refined foods, high in white flour (which is fortified with iron, but not with other trace metals), in sugar and in fat, and drink mostly soft drinks, we may very well be low in trace minerals. Recent work by Colorado pediatricians showed that in Denver some middle-class children may have suffered impaired growth because of an inadequate supply of zinc in the diet. And, of course, iodine deficiency used to be prevalent in many parts of the country—the Ohio Valley, the Great Lakes region, some areas of Texas, the mountain states.

Fluorine is lacking in certain water supplies.

Particularly in areas where the water runs on granite, few minerals are dissolved in it and the water is very soft. It is easier to wash clothes in it but there are some indications that hard water is better for your heart—for reasons we don't understand yet.

In general, the body needs a great variety of the chemical elements, but it needs some of them in much larger amounts than it does others. These "big-quantity" elements are fairly familiar: carbon and hydrogen, for example, which are plentiful in carbohydrates, proteins, and fats. Proteins also contain nitrogen and sulfur. Phosphorous, calcium, and magnesium, as we have seen, are essential to metabolism and to healthy bones. Sodium, potassium, chlorine, and iron are all vital. So are a number of other elements, but in miniscule amounts. Until recently, the quantities of such elements (usually minerals) in our foods and tissues could only be recorded as "traces," thus the name "trace minerals." These (and all are now regarded as essential) microelements are: copper, iodine, zinc, chromium, manganese, fluorine, cobalt, aluminum, bromine, molybdenum, nickel, tin, vanadium, silicon and selenium. Plants require most of them as well (except perhaps iodine and fluorine), and any soil severely depleted would give you a much smaller crop. In many areas of the world, indeed, trace minerals such as molybdenum are included in fertilizer.

Just how small are some of the quantities involved in computing the needs for these minerals and their availability to us in particular foods?

We can do our own measuring of them in fractions of a millionth of a gram! To understand their role, we must picture each cell in our bodies as a complex factory where thousands of chemical reactions go on at the same time to make us the living, breathing, growing, regenerating organisms we are. In an ordinary factory, such chemical reactions could take place only with highly concentrated compounds at high temperatures. In the cells, they occur at body temperature, in watery fluids with enzymes acting as catalysts. These enzymes, composed of complex protein molecules, have the amazing capacity to bring specific molecules to the right position to react at the appropriate moment. Some of these enzymes contain vitamins as part of their own molecules and many do not function except in the presence of the right trace mineral. Without such activators (and each enzyme requires a particular activator), no reaction takes place. If this happens, you may become anemic, or you do not grow; in extreme cases, you may die.

How important are such minerals as copper and zinc?

Copper is essential for the manufacture of hemoglobin. Although it is as vital as iron, the body requires less than a tenth as much. Like iron, copper is almost absent from milk, which is why babies cannot stay on milk alone for too long, even if they are given vitamins. Copper appears in the liver, heart, kidneys, bones, muscles and central nervous system. It is concerned in the formation of brain tissues and in the transport of iron. Particularly good sources of copper are oysters, liver, peas, beans, and whole grain.

Lack of zinc in the diet is believed responsible for the dwarfism observed in some isolated areas in the Middle East.

Besides being necessary to growth, zinc plays a role in the development of sex organs, the manufacture of blood cells, and the healing of wounds and burns. Insulin, the hormone that helps us utilize our blood sugar, requires zinc. Zinc performs a role in the transport of carbon dioxide to the lungs from the tissues and in the utilization of blood glucose. Zinc is common to many foods: meat, fish, eggs, whole grains, vegetables and oysters. The 1974 Recommended Dietary Allowances for the first time set a requirement for zinc: 15 milligrams per day.

If vitamins and minerals are as important as nutritionists insist, why can't I just get a supply of the appropriate capsules and depend on them?

There are two conspicuous and, I hope, convincing reasons why food should be regarded as the nourishment of choice by the human being. One of the things of which my colleagues and I are certain is that nutrition still has its secrets. We must keep prying into them. If the history of the development of our science is a dependable guide, there may be nutrients performing significant duties for us that we have not yet identified. In particular, there may be minerals functioning heroically to our benefit and all unknown to us. If they exist, we are getting them from the varied diet we enjoyably consume. Attempting to depend on "appropriate capsules" might deprive us of substances that we now have and will continue to need. We also need non-nutrients such as fiber.

About a month ago I read that chromium supplements have improved the utilization of sugar in the blood of some diabetics. Since then, I have been trying unsuccessfully to get more information about chromium. Can you help me?

Chromium has an important role in carbohydrate metabolism. It increases the effectiveness of the action of insulin on glucose. Since insulin-dependent diabetics have abnormalities of chromium metabolism, it seemed to be a logical idea to add chromium to their diet. When this was done to a group of them, however, the results were mixed. Only about half showed improvement as measured by glucose tolerance.

Decreased body stores of chromium have been found in diabetics, in women after repeated pregnancies, and as a result of the aging process. But explanations of these phenomena await discovery.

Of particular interest is the observation that the American diet supplies less chromium than those in many parts of the world. Once again, the accusatory finger points at the fact that our diet contains large amounts of refined cereals and sugar. Only minute amounts of chromium are needed on a daily basis. And there is at present no justification for taking a chromium-containing mineral supplement, as some have suggested, especially as we do not know enough about the different degrees of availability to the body of various chromium-containing substances. However, I do think it is a good idea to include plenty of chromium-containing foods, particularly whole grains as well as fruits and vegetables, in your diet. An occasional serving of liver or kidneys is also a good practice.

Do you consider fluorine one of the trace elements or do you lump it with such minerals as calcium, iron and sodium?

Fluorine, as fluoride, is one of the minerals we need in preposterously small quantities, but require just as urgently as we do those that are necessary in greater amounts. By now, almost everyone must know that fluoride contributes to the growth of strong, decay-resistant teeth. In some fortunate communities, it is present in the drinking water. Where it isn't, it is added to the water in small quantities. Some people quibble about this, protesting that fluoride is served, willy nilly, to all when those who immediately benefit are the young. These good folk forget that the youngsters who have received fluoride will become adults with better teeth. There is also suggestive evidence, some of it obtained in studies conducted by Harvard scientists, which indicates that elderly people who have consumed fluoridated water all their lives are less likely to develop osteoporosis (due to loss of calcium from their bones) and suffer less from hip and other fractures.

The amount of fluoride in foods varies with the water where the foods are raised. In Lubbock, Texas, the water contains about 3.8 milligrams of fluoride per liter, while in Yellow Springs, Ohio, the amount of fluoride is only a tenth of a milligram per liter of water. Recent studies with rats show that fluoride is actually necessary for the proper growth of the animal, and is thus in every sense of the term a required mineral. The Food and Nutrition Board of the National Research Council now classifies fluoride as an essential nutrient.

It has astonished me to hear that such items as aluminum and tin are consumed regularly by all of us and may be important to our health. Are there similarly astonishing substances that we eat and need?

It all depends on your level of astonishment. We are not certain that aluminum is essential for man, but it probably is. A deficiency of tin has held back the growth of experimental animals. And nickel seems to be tied to thyroid hormone and epinephrine (adrenalin). It is unlikely that nickel deficiency could occur to anyone on a sound diet.

Here is a little information about several of the minor minerals: Cobalt makes up 4.5 percent of vitamin B_{12}, which protects against pernicious anemia. We do not seem to need cobalt as such, only as a component of vitamin B_{12} which we get from nearly all animal products. The liver and kidneys of ruminants are specially good sources. Yogurt is low in vitamin B_{12}.

We know that plants need boron for growth, but we're uncertain about its importance, if any, to animals and men.

Selenium appears to cooperate with vitamin E in preventing certain muscle defects.

Manganese is needed to activate enzymes which split amino acids off protein, and to obtain energy from the utilization of carbohydrates. The best sources are cereal bran, soybeans, other beans and peas, nuts, tea and coffee.

Cadmium may be essential in tiny amounts and toxic in large ones, but we don't know yet. The same is true of bromine.

Vanadium and silicon are known to be essential for the growth of animals, and vanadium again for their reproduction.

Molybdenum may be significant for the working of a number of enzymes. Molybdenum deficiency has been implicated in certain dental deformities in New Zealand.

2 WEIGHT AND WELL-BEING

7

NUTRITION AND OBESITY: EXERCISE

More Americans are afflicted with obesity than are people of any other country from which we have any dependable accumulation of data. This has been true for a long time and the situation is, apparently, getting worse. Obesity is conspicuously increasing among adolescents, but it is still most prevalent among men and women in their forties and fifties. Among people in their sixties there is less obesity, because so many of its victims have died from diseases of the heart, diabetes, gall bladder diseases, accidents and other untoward events to which the obese are disproportionately subject.

People frequently become obese not because they eat more than thinner people but because they are less active than the slender. This has been observed in all age classes from infancy to the aged. Ancestry plays a part in this.

In the Boston area, we found that 7 percent of the children of thin parents (or at least parents not overweight) are too heavy. If one parent is overweight, the proportion jumps to 40 percent. If both parents are overweight, the proportion of overweight children reaches 80 percent. That heredity is involved is shown by the fact that adopted children, even those adopted from birth, do not show this correlation. This finding has been confirmed by a large-scale study in London, which also showed that naturally acquired children inherited both their body type (size of bones and muscles, general shape of the head, hands, feet and body) and a tendency to overweight. Adopted children showed no such inherited traits or tendencies.

The fact that you may have inherited a tendency to overweight, however, does not necessarily mean you are doomed to be overweight. You still must overeat or underexercise to become overweight. You are just more likely to do these, and thus have to be more watchful—and work harder—if you want to avoid overweight.

Environment, of course, plays a role in the omnipresence of obesity in America. Society demands less activity from more and more people and provides insufficient opportunity for exercise to function as a substitute for the activity the environment once insisted upon.

We are learning more and more about the mechanism in the brain which regulates the sense of hunger and satiety and thus controls caloric intake. We have established that the mechanism just does not operate at very low levels of activity. Unfortunately, this is where more and more of us live!

The fact is that most of the obese can participate in appreciable quantities of regular exercise without increasing their appetites. They do not respond to that increase in exercise by eating enough to prevent the weight loss for which they strive. Indeed, in the course of animal experiments, we learned that rats exercised one or two hours daily ate somewhat *less* than rats which were not exercised at all. Neither we nor my rats were born to be sedentary.

Reducing weight is difficult for almost all people, but there are those who succeed in doing it. The formula is the one here given: *regular exercise and a diet that cuts down on the quantity of food consumed without lessening too much the supply of required nutrients. The best source of a diet is your own physician or a dietitian at the weight-reduction clinic of a large hospital.*

First, I shall discuss the first part of the formula—exercise. Diet is dealt with in the next chapter.

Exercise is very important in weight control. The most widespread fallacy that stands in the way of successful dieting is the belief that food intake alone determines how fat you are.

Your weight, like your bank balance, depends on how much you take out as well as how much you put in. It is far more difficult to lose weight if the only muscles you ever use are the chewing muscles. An hour's walk at 3–4 miles an hour is worth 250 calories if you weigh 150 pounds. This is *half* the caloric deficit you need to have daily if you want to lose one whole pound a week! It is generally easier and far more healthful to lose weight by a combination of calorie reduction and exercise than it is by caloric cutting alone. *So don't forget to step up your activity.*

Although Americans generally have been getting fatter and fatter over the last seventy years, the surprising fact is that people today actually eat less food and get fewer calories than they did in 1900.

The only possible explanation must be inactivity. Today we would label as "moderately active" any neighbor who walks an hour a day, does some gardening, and plays tennis or golf every weekend. But, at the turn of the century, such a man would have been called sedentary.

Possibly the health profession could best serve the population by somehow making us exercise more. But I am convinced that U.S. medicine has yet to recognize fully the formidable health problem caused by the growing physical inactivity (now almost total) of our citizens. Doctors certainly have not come to grips with this problem in their personal lives: I don't know many who have their own daily regimen of exercising. And while they may prescribe more exercise for their patients, they do it without much conviction. They almost never put their recommendations in the form of a detailed program similar, say, to the taking of a drug they might prescribe or even to the dietary schedule established by the dietitians to whom they may refer you.

The main concern, of course, is the connection between the lack of physical activity, the problem of overweight, and the threat of heart disease. (See Chapter 8.)

Men are the major victims. The rate of heart-disease deaths in men and women was about the same at the beginning of the century, but today it is two and a half times as great for males.

Cigarette smoking, diets that are high in fats, high blood

pressure that remains untreated—all these are important elements in the rise of heart trouble. So is physical inactivity, but nobody has yet given enough importance to the element of exercise and the lack of it. Nobody, for instance, has proved in the acceptable, "definitive" scientific fashion that there's any clear connection between exercise and cholesterol. Yet it has been shown that hard, prolonged physical work—at a level probably impossible for us to manage in our urbanized societies —can lower serum cholesterol even among people who eat a high-fat diet.

Lumberjacks in Finland, for example, eat extremely large amounts of food—over 4,700 calories a day, compared to the recommended average of about 2,700 for the adult male American. And almost half of the lumberjacks' diet is fat. But they also engage in hard physical labor for many hours each day. And their blood cholesterol levels have been found to be no higher than those of their average countrymen whose diets consist of fewer calories and a much lower proportion of fat, but who exercise about as much as the typical American male. My own work, with Doctor Daniela Gsell, has shown that Swiss mountaineers, on a diet high in milk, butter and cheese—but with constant day-long exercise—have lower cholesterols than their urbanized brethren who ride cars and streetcars and work at highly sedentary occupations. Mortality from heart disease is very low among mountaineers.

There is other evidence, such as a famous study showing that London bus drivers had a greater rate of heart disease— and more severe disease—than bus conductors. The two groups of men ate essentially identical diets, and the only thing that might account for the difference in heart disease was the conductor's activity. In a double-deck bus a conductor climbs stairs a lot.

"But," you might demand:

"Isn't it really the stress of traffic on the drivers that contributed to the difference?"

Another study suggests that it isn't. A comparison of post office clerks and rural-delivery mailmen revealed that the death rate from heart disease was higher among the clerks than among the mailmen—in spite of all those English dogs! Stress is unlikely to be the critical factor.

Exercise is a vague term. Can you break down exercise into categories and indicate which ones are most suitable for bringing about specific wanted results?

I'll start with what I'll call *moderate exercise.* Some type of physical activity, particularly walking, should be pursued every day for a sufficient time—say, one hour. This activity is essential for controlling weight, especially for people who are mesomorphic or mesomorphic-endomorphic body types, with large skeletons, well-developed muscle structure and a tendency to adiposity or even well-developed fatness.

Limbering, coordinating, and strengthening exercises. Although useful in helping young people to develop physically, and look "fit," these types of exercises are probably of less significance as far as health is concerned.

Constant vigorous physical labor. This kind of activity, obviously incompatible with the mode of employment of most Americans, appears to permit individuals to handle a diet high in saturated fat without the usual increase in serum cholesterol.

Long, hard labor also apparently helps keep the vessels of the heart elastic and open. This in turn helps prevent death from coronary atherosclerosis.

Exercise considerably increasing work of the heart. Exercise properly spaced and sufficiently intense to increase the heart's work load will train the cardiovascular system. The intensity need not approach maximum energy expenditure. Under extreme conditions, the body taps the energy reserved to meet critical needs with little immediate benefit as far as the cardiovascular system is concerned. While this kind of rigorous training is of value to the athlete competing in sprint-type events, it is not indicated for the middle-aged man in need of conditioning.

Is there a close connection between exercise and weight control?

Physical activity is an essential element in appetite and weight control. When you are inactive, the appetite, normally a marvelously precise guide to how much you should eat, no longer functions accurately. In other words, you will eat more than you actually expend, with a corresponding increase in weight.*

The problem of underexercising is particularly significant for children and adolescents. Our studies of overweight schoolchildren in the Boston area show that excessive weight gains usually began in the late fall and winter and almost never during good weather. The overweight children spent strikingly less time in physical activities than their slimmer counterparts. Likewise, we found that on the average the overweight youngsters ate less, not more, than the normal-weight children. So the answer to the weight problems of these children was to increase their exercise rather than decrease their food intake.

Does the same theory apply to adults?

It does, indeed. Our average caloric intake in this country has decreased since 1900, even though our problems of overweight have increased. Of course, since 1900 the automobile has replaced walking, and all sorts of mechanical aids have lightened our toil in the factory, on the farm, and around the home. In the past few years, even such small residual exercises as shifting car gears or pressing the keys of a nonelectric typewriter have been eliminated. And that extra telephone extension in the kitchen may save you steps, but it's worth a few pounds of fat a year.

A pound of fat is the equivalent, on the average, of 3,500 calories. Even a surplus of 100 calories a day—an apple or a serving of potato chips—will grow into 10 pounds of fat a year! But those 100 calories could be used up by walking briskly twenty minutes a day. Remember that exercise does consume an appreciable number of calories, and if you're inactive, you will eat that small but, in the long run, deadly surplus each day. Any exercise done—at however moderate a rate—will bring your appetite back under control if you do it long enough.*

*See Appendix VII.
*See Appendix VIII.

In addition to exercises for a healthier heart and to take off and keep off excess weight, what other benefits does exercise offer?

You may want to develop strength, an important attribute in by-gone days and still a useful asset. Lifting weights or climbing ropes will strengthen your arm and back muscles and help prevent lower back pain later in life. However, before embarking on such strenuous exercises, make sure you're not afflicted with structural weakness, such as a tendency to hernia or slipped disks, and be careful not to overdo.

Then there are exercises to "limber up" and to improve coordination. These make you feel better and improve your looks, grace and ease of movement. Still other exercises will help you keep your stomach flat, a healthful as well as an aesthetically important feature. These types of conditioning exercises often are taught in special-movement exercise or ballet classes, or may be found in any number of exercise books. And each movement of each exercise will take off at least a few of your extra calories, a health by-product for which you may be grateful.

Doesn't participation in team sports provide opportunities for expending calories?

Sometimes very much so. Sometimes not as much as you might think. And other times hardly any at all.

Some team sports that use up a lot of energy are soccer, tennis, hockey and basketball. But some sports, while quite entertaining to players and spectators, do not call for a high, constant disbursement of energy. I would include football and baseball among these. And certain games of skill are great entertainment but no longer physical exercises. If you play golf out of a golf cart, or shoot at clay pigeons on a rifle range, you are not really exercising; you're just playing.

The really important sports are those people can enjoy all their lives. These "lifetime sports" are not team sports; you are unlikely to find twenty-one other people who want to play football just when you do, and it's not easy to get the facilities and the equipment. Nor are track events—except perhaps long-distance running—"lifetime sports." These are, rather, sports such as tennis, squash, hiking, golf, skating, skiing, bicycling, swimming and many water sports including sailing and canoeing.

How highly do you rate such sports as tennis and golf and such individual activities as running?

Tennis, golf (with vigorous walking) and other competitive sports are both good exercise and means of sound mental relaxation because they require almost complete absorption and hence exclusion of the day's worries. Unfortunately few people are able to take part in sports every day. Running is cheap and requires no partner or special equipment. Early in the morning, before breakfast, is a good time of day for running, particularly in suburban neighborhoods. However, it may be more convenient to do it at the end of the day. This is not harmful. In fact, at this time muscles will be somewhat "warmed up" by the normal activities of the day.

Exercise before supper, particularly if vigorous, will usually decrease, rather than increase appetite. There are also psychological advantages of a "break" at the end of the day, whether before supper or just before going to bed. It is often advisable to exercise at a time when you will receive a minimum of attention so that you will not be discouraged by inactive neighbors.

Finally, the conditioning should be gradual so that the increase in physical activity builds on previous performance, producing a steady improvement without excessive effort.

8 NUTRITION AND OBESITY: DIET

Every nutritionist knows—and every dieter must unhappily agree—that crash diets are no good. They're nutritionally unbalanced, they make you weak, irritable and dizzy. Worst of all, from the dieter's viewpoint, they don't work. After the first thrilling plummet of the scales, the pointer inexorably creeps upward again. Looking back, the disappointed dieter knows that all she or he has accomplished is one more useless and frustrating cycle in what I call "the rhythm method of girth control."

Yet people keep on crash-dieting in spite of all the medical warnings and their own experience. Young women and teenage girls, in particular, return again and again to the crash diet, still pursuing the vain vision of instant beauty, since for too many the goal of dieting is rarely better health but greater attractiveness to the opposite sex, something for which they can't bear to wait too long. Few people have the patience for the slow and steady weight loss of sensible dieting. But even that doesn't always work. Why not?

Dieting should work the same way arithmetic works. A pound of fatty tissue is the equivalent in energy of 3,500 calories. Every time you eat 3,500 calories less than you expend— over a period of days—you should use up a pound of fatty tissue. A deficit of 500 calories a day (eating 2,000 and using up 2,500, for instance) should lead to a loss of 1 pound a week, or 52 pounds a year. Double that deficit to 1,000 calories a day, and you can lose 104 pounds a year, surely enough for almost anybody and certainly enough to convince people that crash-dieting isn't even necessary, much less safe.

Yet people keep on "cutting calories," they think, "staying on the diet," they think—and staying the same weight, or practically the same weight, week after week. There is nothing wrong with the arithmetic or with the laws of the conservation of matter and energy.

Where (you have every right to demand) does the problem lie?

It lies in several specific misunderstandings about dieting. There are a number of basic errors to which a dieter can become victim. Let us see how a dieter can avoid them and thus sidestep these traps into which so many well-meaning, determined dieters fall.

Beware of "nonfattening" food. Because, with the possible exception of celery at 7 calories per stalk, there's really no such thing. Too many people believe that there is one big category of food that is nonfattening, another that is fattening. Such people think that a weight-reducing diet consists of a list of foods that are permitted at each meal, and as long as you don't eat the "forbidden" foods, you'll naturally lose weight. Thus, the dieter relieves himself or herself of worrying about arithmetic or the size of portions so long as he or she sticks to the first group—roast beef, yogurt and orange juice—while scrupulously avoiding group two: bread, potatoes, bananas.

This utterly disregards the plain facts: a 3-ounce slice of roast beef (barely enough to decently cover a slice of rye bread) contains 260 calories, plain yogurt 150 calories a cup, and unsweetened orange juice 110 calories a cup. White bread is a mere 60 calories a slice and a fairly large baked potato or a banana only 100—not much more than the dieter's standby, the hard-boiled egg.

What particular moral should we draw from the fact that there is, for all practical purposes, no such thing as nonfattening food?

Calories do count! Those three little words should be recited prayerfully morning, noon and night by everybody who seriously wants to reduce sensibly and successfully.

Few people ever train themselves to look at the difference between a 3-ounce hamburger patty and a 5-ounce patty. If the calorie chart says 310 calories for a hamburger, that's supposed to be that. Yet the larger hamburger contains about 200 more calories, or a total of 510. Just eating one large-size hamburger a day—but counting it as a small one—will make a difference of nearly two pounds of fat a month. A full 8-ounce glass of orange juice instead of a 4-ounce juice glass changes the figure from 55 calories to 110. The hidden surtax on the larger portion can destroy a calorie budget as completely as an obvious food splurge. The *amount* of food as well as the *kind* of food does make a caloric difference.

So *keep your eye on portion size.* And *count every calorie.* Many people forget to take into account "small snacks," especially if they are nibbled over a long period instead of gobbled down in one handful. A cupful of Brazil nuts, unconsciously devoured while watching a football game, doesn't seem worth thinking about. Yet it represents 900 calories! (Peanuts? 805 calories for a mere two fistfuls.)

How much does the fattening ability of food change with different methods of preparing it?

A great deal. The wrongfully called fattening potato contains only about 100 calories, baked or boiled. With salt and pepper, lemon juice, or Worcestershire sauce, it still contains 100 calories. Add one tablespoon of butter or margarine and you double the count. French-fry the potato or mash it with butter and milk, and you've pushed the total to 250. And, if you're addicted to hash-brown potatoes, you should know you're absorbing at least 470 calories per cup.

You can similarly double or triple the calorie content of your 80-calorie egg by frying it in generous amounts of butter or fat, or of your 60-calorie slice of bread by loading it with butter and/or jam. (Incidentally, toasting does nothing to calories; it simply drives out the water and changes the color and texture of the bread.)

On the more cheerful side, you can cut the calories in

hamburgers or steaks by cooking them in a nonstick pan, which does not require any lubricating fat, or better still by using a grill that allows appreciable amounts of fat and calories to drip out of the meat. "Cooking lean" is essential.

I have been trying to restrict the amount of saturated fat in my family's diet. I avoid frying with grease and use nonstick cooking utensils to brown meat. I have heard the quality of food is affected by cooking in nonstick pans. Is this true?

Concern over the safety of nonstick cooking ware has been around as long as the nonstick pans themselves. On the basis of the available evidence, it appears that nonstick pans have been demonstrated as safe for ordinary kitchen use. So if nonstick pans help you to pare your family's saturated fat intake to a minimum, by all means continue to use them.

Is it true that protein contains relatively few calories, and that it somehow "burns" fat?

Actually, protein contains about 120 calories per ounce, the same as carbohydrates. (Fats are more costly, about 270 calories an ounce.)

The idea that protein burns fat started out as a misunderstanding of an old laboratory experiment. It showed, indeed, that if a person ate only pure protein for a meal (and egg white is the only thing in nature that comes close to the definition of pure protein), about 30 percent of the energy eaten would be dissipated as heat shortly after the meal. The problem is that if the meal contains any fat or carbohydrates—as all meals do —the effect is cancelled.

Too many dieters also believe that meat is pure protein, and therefore you can eat steak ad infinitum and emerge as slinky as a cougar. In fact, all meat contains fat. A 3-ounce, 310-calorie hamburger contains, on the average, 19 grams of protein (about 80 calories) and 26 grams of fat (about 230 calories). In other words, about three-quarters of the calories in a hamburger come from the fat. Three ounces of sirloin or deboned rib roast contain 20 grams of protein (80 calories) and 20 grams of fat (180 calories). Ham contains even more fat calories in proportion to protein. Of the 340 calories in a slice of ham, only 80 come from the protein, 260 from the fat. *So stop believing that meat equals protein equals few calories.*

This is not to say that many people do not find that it is easier for them to cut down on calories if their diet is fairly high in protein, because many do. But cutting down on carbohydrates and fat, while keeping the diet reasonably high in protein (through the use of cottage cheese, for example), does not preclude cutting down on calories in general, including meat.

Why is it that some people seem to be able to eat all they want without gaining weight?

If you take people of roughly the same general weight and body build who really do take in the same number of calories each day, the only reason Number 1 gains and Number 2 doesn't is that Number 2 works harder or takes more exercise, thus burning up calories.

If gaining and losing weight is as uncomplicated as you make it sound, how come it's so difficult for most of us who are too fat to lose weight and for many of us who are too thin to gain it?

When it comes to what tends to make you eat or stop eating, our knowledge is far less secure. Nutritionists have done a great deal of work in the past twenty years on the mechanisms of hunger and appetite. In my own laboratory, we have helped identify the brain centers that determine when an animal or a person starts or stops eating and we have demonstrated their anatomical connections. We do not know, however, how they are set so as to determine a person's usual weight. It must be related to body type, which, as already noted, is inherited.

Should someone on a reducing diet cut down on the amount of salt and water he consumes?

Attempts to reduce weight by simply cutting down on salt or water are futile. On the other hand, if you are overweight (or even if you are not), it's a good idea to go easy on salt, because people who ingest large amounts appear to be more prone than others to develop high blood pressure. And for some people, particularly middle-aged women, decreasing salt may allow a more regular weight loss by reducing temporary water accumulation. But cutting down on salt will not by itself reduce your weight, unless it happens to make food so unappetizing that you simply eat less. As for water, it's the world's one and only calorie-free fluid.

Are nondairy powdered cream substitutes acceptable on a weight-reducing diet? They're advertised as having only 11 calories per teaspoon.

There are really very few foods that on some basis can't be worked into a reducing diet. Nutritionists, dealing with individual patients, can even work in an occasional serving of strawberry shortcake (on special occasions).

The answer to the question about powdered cream substitutes, however, must be a qualified, a very qualified, "yes." It is true that these products contain only 11 calories per level teaspoon. But, unfortunately, as you can observe any morning at the office coffee break, people rarely use one level teaspoon. In order to lighten the coffee sufficiently, they're likely to use two or more heaping teaspoons. By then, they've added as much as 35 calories which is about the same thing as using three teaspoons of coffee cream.

I may add that these cream substitutes are usually based on coconut oil, which is at least as saturated as the butter fat in cream, so you certainly don't profit much with their use. Palm oil, used in some of the "creamers," is also a saturated fat. Creamers are also devoid of riboflavin (vitamin B_2) and calcium, two good reasons to include whole milk or skim milk in your diet. In fact, if you look at the labels of most of them you will recognize them as foods made entirely of additives!

It seems that nearly everyone I know who's dieting or worrying about his weight is eating yogurt. Is there something magical about yogurt?

There is really nothing magical about yogurt or any other single food that makes it a must on a weight-reduction diet. Yogurt is a perfectly good food. It's made from partially skimmed milk to which nonfat milk solids are added. Plain yogurt contains about 150 calories per cup, while its fruit-flavored cousins contain an average of 250 calories. The extra 100 calories come from the preserves, which provide little but sugar.

If you want to include it in your diet, here are some suggestions: you can buy the plain, unflavored yogurt and add instant coffee or your own fresh fruit. A half of a medium-sized banana, for instance, would add only 60 calories. Not only will you save some calories, but you will be improving the nutritional value of the meal. A sliced peach adds about 40 calories, a cup of strawberries 60 calories. Or if you'd rather have a piece of fruit, say an orange for dessert, try a recipe which yogurt enthusiasts seem to enjoy. Slice some cucumber into the yogurt, and have the orange afterward.

Remember that because yogurt comes in a one-cup (and more recently a 5-ounce) container, which most people regard as a serving, you can certainly add some foods to round out the meal. Start with a glass of tomato juice, followed by a dish of yogurt with cucumbers, vegetable sticks and a few crackers. End with a fruit cup and a couple of cookies for a nutritious low-fat lunch.

> *Could you comment on the calorie and fat content of sour cream?*

Sour cream contains about 30 calories per tablespoon, almost all of them from fat. Since it is a dairy product, it is relatively high in saturated fat and does contain some cholesterol.

If you are interested in cutting down both the fat and the calories, you can substitute plain yogurt or a mixture of sour cream and yogurt. Yogurt contains roughly 9 calories per tablespoon. Mixed with chives and served on a baked potato, it provides quite a good substitute for the higher calorie sour cream.

> *I am aware that you do not favor unusual diets for weight-reduction. Assuming, however, that one goes on a low-carbohydrate diet, eats fewer calories, and succeeds in losing weight, what are the objections to this type of regimen?*

One must first define what you mean by success. If, after having got your weight down to a desirable level, you immediately switched to a more normal eating program and continued to maintain your weight loss, one might be inclined to look more tolerantly at the diet. A number of people do find it easier to lose weight on a diet which has sharply reduced carbohydrates. Unfortunately, such diets are habit forming, and continue to be followed after the weight loss is over (and even after the weight has been regained). In the long run, one of the biggest objections to a low-carbohydrate diet—as well as other unusual diets—is that it does nothing positive to improve poor eating habits. Since such diets become pretty monotonous over a long period of time, few people will stay on them. And, of course, there's the extra fatigue and irritability associated with a low-carbohydrate diet.

The other side of low-carbohydrate diets is a high-fat intake. Since many protein-rich foods contain substantial amounts of fat, you have to expect your fat intake—especially the saturated fat intake—to be higher. This is particularly undesirable for a man or post-menopausal women. Certainly, if you are going to go on a low-carbohydrate (and high-fat) diet, you should have your cholesterol tested every two months or so. If it goes up significantly, stop and go back to a prudent diet. Better still, stay on a prudent diet all along!

Finally, if you are still in doubt, there's also the assault on your pocketbook. A low-carbohydrate diet is an expensive way to lose weight. One simply does not need all that protein for tissue growth and repair. What is not needed is simply broken down and burned for energy. Since ounce for ounce, protein and carbohydrate supply the same number of calories, it's a pretty expensive way to get your quota.

I have a friend who is so fat it's just awful. I keep telling her to go on a diet, but she seems to have so many problems. Are there people who should not try to reduce? People who, no matter how fat they are, would do better to remain fat?

There are, indeed, many people whose hold on emotional stability is most precarious. For some fat people, going along with their fatness may be a kind of valor. For them, a severe reducing program would disturb a pattern of existence whose linkages might be too fragile to withstand it. But these connections may one day become stronger. An understanding physician may be able to help decide if and when the time is ripe for a gentle try at getting the weight down. In the meantime, learn to live with your fat friend. Stop nagging!

What is the easiest food for a dieter to cut down on?

Cut down on sugar. It contains 4 calories per gram, just like other carbohydrates. The consumption of 105 pounds of sugar per American per year is the equivalent of 190,000 calories, or 55 pounds of body fat per year. If this isn't going to be accumulated as extra weight, it has to be burned up somehow. If you cut down your sugar consumption (sugar-containing foods and drinks as well as sugar out of a teaspoon) to half the national average, and assuming that your present sugar intake *is* average, you would lose over 27 pounds in a year.

Do polyunsaturated fats contain any calories?

Yes. There is a hopeless mix-up about the relationship between calories, fat and cholesterol. Somehow, millions of people have the idea that any margarine or oil that is high in polyunsaturated fat (or low in cholesterol) is therefore low in calories. It is certainly desirable to replace saturated fat with polyunsaturated fat in order to keep down cholesterol. But oils —saturated or polyunsaturated—butter and margarine have essentially the exact same calorie content per unit weight of fat.

I'm fatter than most people and I'm older than a lot of people—I've noticed that only lately. I seem to bump into things more than I used to. Chairs, doors, the wall. Do fat people have more accidents?

Unfortunately, yes. The fat person, just because he's fat, has to compete for space with chairs, doors and other things much more often than a slender person. And the burden of fat adds to the problem. It's a constant load to carry, and it robs you of some of your alertness. Age is a factor, too. Older people have more difficulty in getting around. And they have a tendency, too, to clutter their homes with objects that frequently get in their way.

Statistics indicate that fat people not only have more accidents than thin people, but more fatal accidents. For example, compared to the population as a whole, 31 percent more overweight men and 20 percent more overweight women die in automobile accidents. After you get your house cleared out a bit, pay your physician a visit. He may put you on a reducing regimen.

81

Saunas have suddenly become popular in our area. The way I look at it, otherwise sensible people sit around and cook themselves into apparent bliss. It's not for me. But friends tell me that I'm passing up an effortless way to reduce my weight. Will a steam bath really take off weight?

Yes, it will. But the weight the sauna takes away won't stay off; it will go, then come right back. If you weigh yourself before and after sweating out in a sauna, you will find that you weigh a little less at the second weighing.

What happens is that you lose a quantity of water. After all, you have a lot to lose. Up to 65 percent of your body is nothing but water in the first place. And, if the sauna is hot enough and you remain inside long enough, you'll lose a quantity of that water. You'll also be thirsty—enough to drink back much of what you've lost. (And you should drink it, too!)

Losing and gaining weight the water way is an everyday affair. We breathe, we perspire, we urinate. In fact, you lose about two-thirds of a pint of water a day by breathing alone. But what you want is to lose fat, not just lose water for a while.

How often should I weigh myself for better weight control?

Even though you may register some unexplained bumps (some middle-aged women tend to retain water for a while during weight reduction; premenopausal women retain some water every month before menstruation), there is some merit in weighing yourself every day and plotting the weight on a chart (like a fever chart at the hospital). You will find it encouraging to note the steady decline. Incidentally, you will minimize the bumps due to retaining water if you cut down on the salt content of your diet. Good luck!

The other night I went to a popular local restaurant and, attempting to watch my diet, ordered broiled shrimp and a baked potato. But included with my dinner were mushrooms in oil, cheese and crackers, a medium ear of buttered corn, a popover, garlic toast with cheese, sour cream and bacon for the enormous baked potato, and a salad drowning in dressing.

I was appalled at the high caloric "window ornaments" accompanying the four shrimp I received. First, what is the caloric value of all this? Second, is there any hope restaurants can be made more responsive to our diet-conscious society?

It's difficult to estimate calories without knowing the portion size. But a conservative guess is about 1,100 calories for the window ornaments and about 140 for the shrimp. (And that doesn't count the calories in cocktails and dessert!) I'm afraid that expecting restaurants to count calories for us is a hopeless dream. Many American restaurants have built their fame and fortune on quantity and high-caloric gimmickry. For those who eat out only occasionally and have no weight problems, such temptations present only minor difficulties. But if weight is a concern, here are three approaches:

If you're going out in the evening, eat conservatively all day.

Be selective in choosing extras.

Eat reasonable servings; there's no reason to feel bound to clean your plate. It may be a waste not to finish the portion served, but it's a greater evil to accumulate extra fat around your waist or in your arteries.

For many business men and women who almost daily eat in restaurants, indiscretion can become the parent of obesity. Your discretion, incidentally, in ordering broiled shrimp instead of an 8-ounce tenderloin steak netted you a savings of 250 calories.

You often refer to the number of calories in a 3-ounce hamburger or a 4-ounce piece of steak, but how does the ordinary person estimate portion sizes with any degree of accuracy?

Assessing portion size is one of the most critical and most difficult aspects of successful dieting, and meats are probably the hardest foods to judge.

It is, of course, possible to buy a small, inexpensive scale to weigh servings of meat and other foods. But there are other methods of estimating portion sizes. A pound of pork chops or lamb chops with relatively large amounts of bone and fat yields between 5 and 7 ounces of lean meat. If you had three chops in the pound, each would yield about 2 ounces of lean meat. The same rule applies to rib, sirloin or porterhouse steak with the bone in—each pound yielding about 6 ounces of well-trimmed lean. And if you're dieting, lean is what you're after. A pound of raw hamburger provides between 9 and 13 ounces of cooked meat. So if you make four hamburgers out of the pound, each will weigh a little less than 3 ounces. This hamburger, incidentally, in a restaurant, would be about 3 inches in diameter and an inch thick. In estimating sliced, cooked meat, a piece approximately 4 inches by 3 inches cut 1 inch thick weighs about 3½ ounces.

> *You said there could be as much as a 100-calorie difference in 3-ounce hamburgers, depending on whether they were made from regular ground meats or from very lean cuts. How does this information relate to trimmed and untrimmed cuts of meat?*

Fats are truly the caloric powerhouse of the diet. Gram for gram, they supply more than twice as many calories as do carbohydrates or proteins. Therefore, lean, well-trimmed meat contains far fewer calories than the same amount of fat-marbled meat.

A relatively fat-laden roast contains 375 calories in a 3-ounce portion, or 205 calories trimmed. A 3-ounce portion of sirloin steak supplies 330 calories if both the fat and lean are eaten, but merely 170 calories if 3 ounces of only lean are eaten. So, if you're in the habit of eating a 5-ounce portion of meat, fat and all, for dinner, and you're interested in cutting down on both calories and fat, simply substitute lean, well-trimmed meat. You will save an average of 225 calories a day, or enough to lose a half-pound a week, without cutting down on your food by a single bite. And, besides, it's better for your heart!

> *I really enjoy cooking, but am also trying to lose weight. Can you tell me how I go about estimating the caloric value of some of the concoctions I create myself?*

Take your recipe for Italian tomato sauce, for example. The recipe, let's say, makes 6 cups of sauce containing 2 onions (80 calories), 3½ cups of canned tomatoes (175 calories), 3 tablespoons of oil (375 calories) and 2 cans of tomato paste (275 calories). Add it all up, divide by 6 and you get 150 calories per cup. If you make sauce with meat, add ½ pound ground beef, browned and drained. This gives you about 6 ounces of cooked meat (490 calories) and raises the caloric value to 230 per cup.

You can reduce the number of calories in a variety of ways. One of the best is to lower the amount of fat. A recipe frequently calls for as much as four tablespoons of oil or fat when two would do. The caloric content is thus effortlessly reduced by 250.

I have recently gone on a diet and am determined to lose weight. I decided to get a good calorie chart but, after comparing a few, I find considerable variation for specific foods. Why is this?

There are a host of reasons for the stated variations in the caloric content of what seems to be a fairly uncomplicated food. These include size of portion described, difference in preparation or recipe, and the relative leanness of meat cuts.

To illustrate the first point—portion size—let's take a grapefruit. In two technical publications widely used by nutritionists, there is a difference of 15 calories. One uses a grapefruit 4 inches in diameter, the other a 4¼-inch grapefruit.

This really need not be a problem since a 15-calorie difference is of little significance for your purposes. This level of accuracy can be achieved in a metabolic research ward, but certainly not in your kitchen.

Variations in methods of preparing food present different problems. Obviously, a broiled chicken leg will have fewer calories than one browned in oil.

So find yourself a good, comprehensive calorie chart. Read carefully how the food is described (a fryer chicken leg is substantially smaller than a roaster leg) and prepared. Let's face it, a breaded veal cutlet is a far cry from a slice of roast veal.

9

NUTRITION AND OBESITY: LIQUID CALORIES

A tribe in Africa long maintained a strong ascendency over nearby tribes simply by convincing their neighbors that they (the convincers) could, through supernatural powers, live indefinitely without food. Their secret was simple: they didn't eat, at least for long periods. But they did drink large amounts of whole milk, the juices of tropical fruits, and beef blood (their chief wealth is cattle, which they rarely slaughter but which they milk and bleed). Their ignorant neighbors, not recognizing that nourishment can be derived from liquids, viewed this practice with awe and acknowledged the supernatural nature of the false fasters.

Before we cluck sadly at such innocence, let's look at our own assumptions as hot weather comes on and tinkling ice cubes and frosted glasses are the order of the day. A grand time for dieters, we think: since it's too hot to eat, we can quench thirst and shed pounds at the same time avoiding all those nasty calories in solid foods. Thus we sophisticated Americans have not advanced much beyond those deceived Africans and not as far as their deceivers in this aspect of nutritional understanding.

I cannot state too strongly that in the summer you will feel most comfortable and function best if you drink enough fluid
and replace fluid losses as you perspire. Unless you are very

suddenly exposed to heat or unless you are exposed to furnace-like temperatures, your body will rapidly adjust itself to conserve salt and you do not need salt tablets (which often cause intense cramps). At most, if you are very active physically in extreme heat, you may salt your food a little more. If you must watch your calories, however, your drinking choice is limited. Tomato juice is good, or you may learn to prefer lime or lemon juice or become adjusted to diluting fruit juice more than you do presently. Iced (light) tea with lemon, not sugar, is low in calories. And don't forget water—which is light, healthful, refreshing and absolutely calorie-free.

Though anxious to reduce our weight and improve our figures, we often act as though no liquid could possibly contain many calories. We have been encouraged in that belief by fads like the "drinking man's diet" or by attending to old wives' tales such as the fiction that beer is fattening but whiskey (or any other hard liquor) isn't. The mistaken belief that alcoholic beverages are low-cal is extended indiscriminately to soft drinks, fruit juices, sometimes milk and milk drinks. This can be costly.

Just how many calories are there in soft drinks?

Ordinarily soft drinks contribute calories (from sugar, as many alcoholic beverages also do) without any other nutrient. The popular varieties of cola beverages, whatever their flavor, vary between 100 and 120 calories per cup. Ginger ale supplies about 80. Gatorade has 40 calories per 8-ounce glass. Since the ban on cyclamates, most low-calorie drinks have used saccharin with a little sugar to mask the bitter aftertaste of that crystalline compound. The amount of sugar used is not revealed on the label, and I cannot, therefore, give the correct figures.

And what are the caloric contents of fruit juice and tomato juice?

Orange juice, a good source of vitamin C and potassium, contains 110 calories per 8-ounce cup (or glass), if it is fresh or canned and unsweetened, 135 if canned and sweetened. A 6-ounce can of frozen orange-juice concentrate, which, diluted, translates into three 8-ounce glasses, has 300 calories, and this much is awfully easy to consume on a hot afternoon. A glass of fresh lime juice contains 60 calories, just a little over half the amount in orange juice. Grape juice, by contrast, is high: 170 calories for the same volume. A glass of fresh grapefruit juice is worth 90 calories; the same volume of sweetened juice goes up to 130. Concentrated frozen grape juice contains 300 calories per 6 fluid ounces (three glasses), the same as orange juice. The best caloric bargain is tomato juice, only 50 calories a glass.

How about the calories in milk and milk beverages?

Milk contains a variable number of calories, depending on its fat content. One cup of whole milk, which is 3.5 percent fat, has 165 calories, skim milk and buttermilk about half that much (85–90 calories per cup). Malted milk drinks contain 280 calories per cup, chocolate-flavored milk 185. The caloric content of milkshakes varies, of course, with the amount of syrup and ice cream used in them. If you feel you simply must have a milkshake, have one, but use skim milk instead of whole. You'll be saving calories.

Everybody knows about the physiological phenomenon called the "beer-belly." How many calories are there in beer, ale and stout?

In beer, ale and stout, calories come from two sources: alcohol and some residual, unfermented carbohydrate. Beer and stout have a higher content of carbohydrate than "light" ale and lager. The color of the dark beer and stout is related to the temperature at which the fermentation process has been stopped: because of greater heat, they are caramelized and acquire a brown color not necessarily related to the caloric content.

Alcohol contains 7 calories per gram. The alcoholic content of beer, ale and stout varies between 3 and 7 percent. An 8-ounce glass of light 4-percent ale contains about 100 calories. This can go up to 200 calories in very strong beer or stout, and the calories add up quickly.

What quantities of calories are in the many and different products of the vintner?

Here, again, calories come from two sources: the alcohol and the sugar. In dry wine, the alcohol contributes almost all the calories. In sweet wines, the sugar content is added. French and German wines have an alcoholic content that varies from 8.5 to 10 percent. American wines have a higher one, usually over 11 percent. Four ounces of dry French wine, with an average of 9 percent alcohol, usually contain 70 to 85 calories; U.S. dry wines, with 12 percent alcohol, 100 calories. Fortified wines, such as sherry and port, have alcohol and sugar added. The alcohol concentration may go to 20 percent, and a sweet sherry and a good ruby port may have over 200 calories in a 4-ounce glass.

How many calories are there in cocktails, sweet liqueurs and spirits?

In cocktails and sweet liqueurs, once again calories come from alcohol and from sugar, but with the great bulk of the calories coming from the alcohol. The difference in caloric content between a Manhattan, an Old Fashioned, and a Martini is negligible. If the "dry" Martini is made with much gin or vodka and only traces of vermouth, the caloric content will be higher than in the sweeter alternatives. These drinks can range from 160 to 200 calories per 2 ounces. Grasshoppers and Brandy Alexanders may go as high as 300. Sweet liqueurs contain 100 calories or more per ounce. Gin, rum, Scotch, and Irish rye are usually 80 proof, which is equivalent to 40 percent alcohol. A shot glass, or 1½ ounces, of whiskey contains about 110 calories.

How do mixers affect the calorie count of alcoholic drinks?

The minute you add anything—except water or club soda —to the alcohol that's the base of your highball, up go the calories. Quinine water contains a relatively moderate 88 calories per 8-ounce glass, bitter lemon or orange go up to 125. Depending on the quantity of whiskey you pour and which mixer you use, a highball (1½ ounces whiskey and the rest water) can run from 110 calories to (two shots of whiskey and a mixture of bitter lemon) 275 calories.

In the report of the White House Conference on Food, Nutrition and Health of which you were chairman, a panel concerned with "Adults in an Affluent Society" said, "Alcohol now provides an average ranging from 10 percent to

20 percent of the total calories consumed by adult North Americans. Although rich in calories, alcoholic beverages are almost devoid of all known essential food factors and vitamins." Then the panel proposed "research with the aim of exploring the feasibility of supplementing commercially available alcoholic beverages with additional nutrients." How is that research coming along? How soon may we look forward to advertised assurances that there's "niacin in your nightcap" or "vitamins in your vodka"?

This proposal is considerably less off-beat than it may appear to be. When the intake of alcohol in any form is allowed to cut into the consumption of necessary food, there is a strong likelihood of the development of serious deficiencies in needed nutrients. When this continues for a long time, the drinker not only damages his health, he endangers his life. I know of no research of the type the panel proposed now going on.

I may add that even though it would make a lot of medical sense to add vitamin B_1 to alcoholic beverages (to prevent "alcoholic beriberi" and its attendant "beriberi heart"), most health authorities would oppose this. They are afraid that such enrichment procedures would encourage alcoholics to drink more because they would feel protected by the addition of nutrients to their favorite form of empty calories.

The scientists have a nightmare which pictures Joe, in his T-shirt, steadily imbibing in front of the TV set. His wife, Jane, tries to get him to come and have dinner and he is saying: "Jane, don't bug me. You take your vitamins your way. I take them my way." Whether this vision of horror would, in fact, come about has never been tested.

What is the story about calories in coffee? I thought coffee was calorie-free, but I notice that the label on the coffee I regularly use states it does have a few calories.

Don't worry about the calories in a cup of coffee. Black coffee contains at most 5 calories per cup, an insignificant amount compared to the 15 to 25 calories per teaspoon of sugar and the 30 calories in a tablespoon of cream. It would take at least ten cups of black coffee just to equal the calories in a chocolate chip cookie, or more than fifteen cups to equal those in a 6-ounce glass of cola, or about thirty cups to equal those in a vanilla ice cream cone. Drinking too much black coffee may be bad for you, but not because of the calories in it.

10 DO YOU WANT TO GAIN POUNDS?

Underweight (roughly defined as being 10 to 20 pounds under ideal weight for height and bone structure) is believed to be considerably less common in the United States than overweight. Whereas the most frequent estimate—with which I concur—of the percentage of overweight people in this country is about 35, I cannot recall an estimate of the percentage of underweight that is higher than a few percent.

Humans become underweight when they take in fewer calories than they use up in activity. And they remain underweight when they do not achieve an intake sufficient to reach a higher weight and stay in balance there.

The determination of whether a person is underweight, the search for the causes of the condition, and the prescription for what should be done about it are, of course, a matter for the physician.

Many factors can cause people to lose weight without intending too. Among them are glandular disorders of various sorts and several diseases. When none of these conditions exists, the problem of chronic underweight is found to be in the same departments where the problem of overweight is discovered, those that cover activity and nutrition.

Poverty may have a lot to do with underweight. So may ignorance. So may isolation or, in the cases of the aged and the young, neglect. The victim of underweight may be a meal-misser. Or he or she doesn't get sufficient rest. Frequently this latter condition is brought about not by overexertion but by not getting enough exercise to assure a good night's sleep. The tossing and turning that accompany insomnia may use up significant numbers of calories.

Most physicians advise their underweight patients to follow an appropriate diet that is calorically larger than has prevailed. They may also prescribe nourishing snacks and supplements of the vitamins and minerals such as iron. And it is likely that they will urge regular exercise of a sort suitable to each patient's age, occupation, health and temperament.

One of the most serious conditions associated with underweight is one most frequently found in young women. It is called "anorexia nervosa," a state in which the victim professes no hunger for food in general nor appetite for any food in particular. Sometimes the patient makes herself vomit what little she has eaten. What occurs is a period of self-initiated and self-continued starvation. If this goes on long enough, the result is, of course, death. The problem is a difficult psychiatric one.

In contrast to this harsh and, blessedly, uncommon disease, there are tens of thousands of people trying to *gain* weight. And theirs is a lonely struggle. Swimming against the current as they do—clearly outnumbered by the millions of Americans struggling to *lose* weight—they can expect little help from the media or from the merchants of facile cures. And yet their desire to alter their body image is just as intense, and sometimes just as desperate, as that of their overweight neighbors.

It has been said that within any obese person there is a thin man or woman trying to get out. But the thin person has no such obvious imagery and thus lacks any idea of what his or her "perfected" body should look like. And, as we shall see, the problem of congenitally thin persons trying to gain weight seems infinitely harder than that of heavy people trying to lose (at least temporarily) excess pounds.

First, the mandatory question:

Who are these unhappy thin people, and just why do they want to gain weight?

Over the years, I've observed a marked difference in attitude and expectations between thin men and thin women.

Young men who want to gain weight are usually seventeen to twenty-five years old. They have looked at themselves in the mirror and decided that their excessive slimness makes them appear young, weak, and somehow negligible in the eyes of the opposite sex. Their shoulders are narrow, their arms are stick-like, without apparent muscles. Their legs, drooping out of tennis shorts or swimming trunks, look frail and pathetic. These young men feel that if they could project an image of protective strength they would be more attractive to the shapely, graceful girls they sit by in classrooms or watch playing volleyball or admire at the beach. The thin men observe the casual, easy relationships the more muscular types have with girls, and they feel doubly left out. In their own eyes, they are the 98- or maybe 118-pound weaklings who get sand kicked in their faces by the "heavies" they would like so much to emulate.

They generally work hard at gaining weight. They lift barbells. They buy "isometric" exercise machines. They drink "body-building" liquid diets. They force themselves to eat at least part of servings of rich desserts. And nothing seems to help.

In what way are the problems of underweight young women different from those of underweight young men?

Young women who are underweight—and concerned about it—are not primarily interested in becoming heavier "all over," though many would accept some general inflation if this were the only way to acquire more weight where they specifically want it.

For the most part, these girls are preoccupied with their uncurved, boylike bodies, even though they appear to be the ideal of so many women's fashion designers. They would like to have rounder arms, somewhat rounder thighs, certainly a little more of a derrière and, of course, a much bustier chest. They watch with anxiety the interest of their male contemporaries in deep cleavages and rounded hips and they despair of ever really engaging and holding the passionate interest of any man.

Just as so many overweight girls feel that success, love and all the good things of life would come to them if only they could lose weight, the thin, flat-chested girls are convinced that if they could put a few pounds on the more strategic points of their bodies, their dreams could come true. They usually try to eat their way to their standard of excellence through heavy cream, milkshakes and frequent "high-caloric" snacks which, when measured, turn out to be pitiably small. For those of us who love young people, the pathos of these inadequate self-images, both for boys and girls, is almost heartbreaking.

Can these young men and women be helped very much?

First, let us recognize that from the viewpoint of *physical health,* they don't really need help. When they consult a physician or a nutritionist, they ordinarily say they would like to gain weight because they think the added pounds would make them "feel" better.

There is little scientific basis for believing that this is literally true. All the data we have from insurance statistics agree that the thinnest people live longest and are least affected by the so-called degenerative diseases—heart, liver, and kidney disorders and diabetes. They even seem to have fewer accidents. Cancer does not follow this pattern. Overall, weight does not seem to be a factor either way, although with some types of malignancies there may be a correlation with overweight.

An intriguing exception is suicide: the overweight are less likely to kill themselves than are their thinner brethren. But, all in all, thinness, even extreme thinness, has an excellent prognosis unless, of course, it is caused by disease. If you're interested in living a long life, thinness is to be prized.

There is, of course, little comfort in this for the troubled, lonely young person who's dissatisfied with his or her body and who's anxious to present a more attractive appearance to the opposite sex. One wants to help these unhappy people, not for reasons of their bodily health or to make them better physically; you want them to be more secure and accept themselves better.

But the assistance you offer is very unlike the kind of help they seek, isn't it?

Well, when it comes to aiding them to gain weight, there is little that can be done. In this particular, the very thin are, as far as a solution to their problem is concerned, very like the very fat, except more so.

The very fat can lose weight if they are placed on a low-calorie diet—even if you have to lock them up in a hospital room to do it. The very thin—by that I mean not just ordinarily thin, but *very* thin—are almost impossible to fatten up. They frequently tell you that they are thin in spite of (to listen to them) gargantuan meals. But when you measure their overall intake in the course of a day, it is often quite small.

What they really mean when they tell you they eat "a lot" is that they force themselves to eat even when they are not hungry. In much the same manner, people who are overweight will insist, with equal sincerity, that they eat "like a bird." What they are really saying is that they eat far less than they could eat or would like to eat.

Here is something that might help certain of the very thin to pick up a few pounds: since they are often quite active they might increase their weight if they can cut down on their physical activity without cutting down on their food intake.

Is it possible that the tendency to extreme thinness might involve an inherited factor and thus be strongly resistant to correction?

It is indeed. There does seem to be a genetic determination of thinness—probably a lack of adipose cells (those specialized in accumulating fat). Most individuals have "fat depots" of these cells, grouped under the skin in specific areas: on the abdomen, around the kidneys, under the chin. These can fill up with fat if a person eats more calories than are expended. One pound of fat, on the average, accumulates every time you have eaten 3,500 more calories than you have expended. But if you don't have the adipose cells, you obviously can't fill them.

Our work at Harvard's Nutrition Department suggests that persons with these very limited fat depots are also people with sudden and complete feelings of satiety. Unlike most of us, who can usually be persuaded to have a little more of a favorite dish, these constitutionally thin people stop feeling hungry quite abruptly and would gag at another mouthful.

An interesting fact, discovered by Dr. C. C. Seltzer and me a few years ago, is that these people are generally ectomorphs, a body type having a slender, elongated skeleton, narrow hands and feet, long fingers and toes. Dr. Seltzer, a noted physical anthropologist, cautions that these permanently thin ectomorphs should not be confused with what he calls "late-blooming endomorphs." The latter, though often self-conscious because of their thinness when very young and actively trying then to gain weight, have an entirely different body type that blossoms out in early middle age in spreading adiposity. They never showed the elongated skeleton of the ectomorphs; they simply had inactive or empty depot fat cells. And, as their thirties roll on, their potentially ample fat cells fill up—to the extent that they remember with melancholy the time when they wanted to gain weight.

The way you tell it, the whole problem of weight control sounds extremely complex. Is that the actual situation?

It is, and the inability of the constitutionally very thin to gain weight is an excellent example. Calories *do* count, and anyone who says they don't and that you can eat as much as you want without gaining weight as long as the calories come exclusively from meat, or martinis, or rice, or whatever, is practicing quackery.

On the other hand, to reaffirm this basic law of nature does not mean that anyone can easily gain or lose weight simply by deciding to eat more or less. Very complex mechanisms regulate food intake, spontaneous activity and the rate of fat synthesis or utilization. And the difficulty—indeed, the near impossibility—for many very thin people to gain weight, even temporarily, is a parallel of the difficulty that many fat people have in losing weight, at least permanently.

But what specifically should a thin person who wants to gain weight do about it?

The best advice for very thin people is, I believe, first to have a thorough checkup to make sure their thinness is not associated with a chronic disease—diabetes, tuberculosis, anemia or some other condition—which needs to be diagnosed and treated. On confirmation that they are healthy, the best course is to forget about trying to gain weight and concentrate on two targets.

First, fitness: they will look far better if they appear exercised, with a healthy outdoor tan and good posture. (Posture is particularly important—so many tall, thin people try to look shorter and heavier by stooping. Of course, all they accomplish is potential back problems and a far less attractive image!)

Second, fashion: the right clothes, the right hairdo and makeup for women, the right haircut for men will make a considerable difference in their appearance—which is their main worry. They must learn to turn their slimness into an asset. After all, what is more attractive than a slim waist, set off by wearing the right kind of stripes or figured shirts or dresses? If a young woman is really self-conscious about a flat chest, she can add natural-looking curves with a padded bra. Professional models have learned to make their reed-like figures their greatest asset, and many of their techniques can be profitably adopted by thin people.

So get some exercise and plenty of rest. Stop smoking cigarettes if you are a smoker. And rejoice in the knowledge that you can eat such high caloric delicacies as pâté de foie gras, eggnog and fruit cake.

You always have lots of good information for people with a problem of excess weight. I'm at the other extreme. I simply can't gain weight. My husband says I'm too skinny, but I've always been very thin. Is there anything I can do about this?

Your husband apparently welcomed your skinniness when he married you, and probably that's the way he'll have to accept you always! But if you think you'd like to go all-out and try to gain some weight for purely cosmetic purposes, you might begin by paying more attention to snacks. A small midmorning snack, one in midafternoon and a third before bed can substantially expand your daily caloric intake. Eat snacks at times that don't spoil your appetite for meals, however. My suggestions are cookies, half a sandwich and a glass of milk, cheese and crackers with juice, a cup of soup, fruit or maybe even a dish of yogurt.

NEWCOMERS AND TODDLERS

Whenever our press, weary of reporting on bombings, crime rates and unemployment statistics, looks for something more cheerful to convey to the American public, we are told that our children are getting taller. And indeed they are: in Boston, the average fourteen-year-old is six inches taller than his counterpart of a hundred years ago. Over 25 percent of our young men are more than six feet tall, as compared with 4 percent in 1900.

But, alas, there is another altered physical characteristic, rarely commented upon: Americans are getting fatter even faster than they are getting taller. Our Boston fourteen-year-old is not only taller, he is also over thirty pounds heavier than his 1870s' model.

From 1940 to 1960, the average weight of American men went up ten pounds. And the increase is accelerating, with recent statistics of the U. S. Public Health Service indicating that over half of adult men are overweight! Forty percent of adult American women also weigh more than is conducive to greatest longevity.

In suburban Boston schools, the proportion of obese children has grown in twenty years from 12 to 20 percent. One reason for this increased prevalence of overweight is obviously the growing physical inactivity of our population and, in particular, of our children. A number of years ago, I showed first in experimental animals, then in people of various ages, that while appetite is a fairly good guide to the amount of food needed by active subjects, it is not a reliable measure for inactive ones.

When daily exercise is minimal, most children and adults eat more than they need. In other words, if you walk ten miles during the day you will automatically be hungrier than if you walk two miles. But it does not follow that if you don't walk at all you will want to eat less than if you walk two miles. You will probably eat as much—and you will get fatter.

We also found that individuals who are endowed with a large bone and muscle mass (the type physical anthropologists call mesomorphs) need to exercise more than ectomorphs (elongated types with narrow hands and feet) to reach the point at which their appetites automatically dictate the right amount of food for them to eat.

In a number of studies, stretching over twenty years, we showed that the big difference between most overweight children and adolescents and their thin contemporaries was not that the overweight youngsters eat more, but that they exercise far less than other children who are of normal weight.

What factors have brought about the current lack of physical activity among the young?

Unfortunately, a number of school systems have dropped the requirement for even the sketchy physical-exercise program once offered to all students. With the growing affluence of the middle class, more and more American families own a second —and a third—car. This means that if by some chance children don't ride a school bus, Mother drives them to school. And if the youngsters are old enough, they will drive themselves. In a number of urban schools, with land at a high premium, school committees have converted playground areas into student parking lots!

The effect of the elimination of walking is compounded by the hours spent daily in front of the television set. While every educator in America worries about exposing children's impressionable minds to hours of mediocre fare, I worry also about the effect on their bodies.

A recent large-scale study discloses that preschool children watch TV an average of five hours a day. Our studies of children's schedules show that a great deal of this "viewing" (and sitting) time has replaced playing time—active games in the backyard or neighborhood playground. This drastic curtailment of physical activity has been both so gradual and so nearly universal that most parents seem unaware of it. But it shows up in the lack of fitness and the overweight of too many children.

At what stage in a child's life does this overweight commence?

A number of nutritionists and pediatricians are beginning to show deep concern over the possibility that we are overfeeding babies in a way that will produce an enormous proportion of fat babies and also actually modify their anatomy so that they will be prone to obesity for the rest of their lives!

Specifically, we feel that the recent practice of giving babies not only high-caloric formulas but baby foods that contain many more calories than does mother's milk may lead them to eat more than they need for harmonious growth. This practice also may induce the formation of additional fat cells which *all their lives* will greedily sop up nutrients from their blood, leading them to over-eat and become excessively fat.

Will you explain how this process seems to work?

You must understand a little basic physiology, but let me reassure you, it need not be too technical. First, the mechanism of appetite in newborn infants is probably different from that in older children and adults. Humans have an automatic "calorie counter" in the hypothalamus, the part of the brain that regulates a number of basic body functions such as temperature control. The "satiety" centers of the hypothalamus send special messages to other parts of the brain to turn off your desire to eat when you have had enough calories. The volume of the food seems far less important than the calorie content.

Laboratory experiments show that most adults can adjust almost instantaneously to changes in caloric density. You'll stop after eating a small piece of calorie-rich cheesecake, whereas you might consume a larger portion of a food with more dilute calories. Actual "fullness" of the stomach has little lasting effect and is not the reason why you stop eating. In fact, studies show that even removal of part of the stomach (in cancer or ulcer operations) has slight bearing on the amount of food consumed in the course of a day. It just leads to consumption of a larger number of smaller meals.

Does this "calorie-counter" work the same way in infants that it does in adults?

By contrast, our studies at Harvard and those of Gordon Kennedy at Cambridge University in England show that this hypothalamic system is not yet fully operating in very young animals, and that babies probably stop eating because they are literally full. Most babies cannot be overfed by parents who try to make them consume a larger *volume* of milk or formula than they want. A baby will turn his head away and close his mouth or, if forced to ingest extra milk, will regurgitate it immediately. (An old pediatric adage is that it's impossible to overfeed a breast-fed baby.)

However, babies may have very little defense against being fed an overconcentrated diet. For eons, young infants have consumed mostly breast milk—with 67 calories per 100 milliliters. Solid and semisolid foods fed to infants may contain up to 200 calories per 100 milliliters. Prepared baby foods, such as egg yolk, meats, cereals, desserts, some meat dinners, and most fruits (which often have considerable added sugar) contain more calories per unit than breast milk, in many cases two to three times as much!

Young infants may not be able to handle such high concentrations—and the younger they are, the less they're able to adjust. Premature infants seem to be the least capable of adjusting to greater variations in calorie content.

Is there some difference in the behavior of cells in young infants that can work in favor of the accumulation of fat?

In the young infant, the fat cells are still multiplying. In older children and adults, the number of fat cells seems fixed, like that of the brain and nerve cells. Getting fat simply means that you are filling up these specialized "reservoir" cells with fat. But in infants these cells are still dividing. A number of experiments—conducted at Cambridge University by Dr. R. A. McCance and Dr. Elsie Widdowson, and at Rockefeller University by Dr. Jules Hirsch—have demonstrated that overfeeding very young animals leads to the development of extra fat cells, which presumably persist through life.

And studies have repeatedly shown that obesity is most stubborn when it has occurred early in life. Too many mothers "jump the gun" with solid foods. While well-informed pediatricians nowadays usually do not prescribe solid foods before the age of three months, we find that a great many young mothers believe that the use of such foods is some sort of status symbol, something like baby taking that first step or getting a first tooth. As a result, they start babies on solid foods at two months, or sometimes as early as six weeks.

What dangerous mistake do new mothers frequently make?

Many of them, obsessed by weight as the only measure of growth (unfortunately, they don't routinely measure the length of their babies), often rejoice at what is, in fact, evidence of overfattening. Yet they should be particularly wary, if (a) a number of their own or their husband's relatives are overweight; (b) the baby looks fat, or at least is a "broad" rather than a "long" baby; or (c) the baby is unusually inactive.

All too often, mothers forget that babies, too, need exercise. They may seem to be little bundles of activity, but in reality, too many babies spend most of their waking hours confined in playpens, strollers, or car seats, rather than exploring their worlds.

In our studies, all these traits are associated with an above-average risk of obesity, which may be lifelong.

What specific suggestions do you believe an alert pediatrician would probably make to the mother of such an obesity-threatened infant?

Your pediatrician might well suggest the following:

Wait until the baby is four to six months old before introducing solid foods. Cereals with fruit and strained foods such as egg yolk, meats, desserts and high-meat dinners, which are high in calories, may be introduced late and used sparingly. Preference may be given to relatively low-calorie foods, such as plain baby cereals in boxes dinners and vegetables (with no starch or sugar added). Now that baby foods have nutritional labeling you can compare the calories and the nutrients in different foods.

Give unsweetened juices (and water!) as an alternative to milk for slaking thirst, especially during hot weather when children drink more.

Recheck the baby's formula after a few weeks to insure that it is not too rich. If your baby is gaining too much weight, your doctor may dilute the formula or switch to skim milk.

Remember, children have individual differences in their eating behavior and physical development. There is no point in pushing a susceptible baby into the health risk of being too fat.

From more experienced mothers-to-be I receive a lot of conflicting instruction about the proper amount of weight gain during pregnancy. What do you recommend?

A pregnant woman should put on two or three pounds a month during her pregnancy. That means she should gain not less than eighteen pounds and not much over thirty. If she's very thin, she can afford to put on more weight than average, say twenty-four to thirty pounds. If she's heavy to start, she should try to gain no more than eighteen to twenty-four pounds.

While pregnant, a woman is less active, especially in the last three months. She won't need too many extra calories to gain the needed weight. Instead of adding new foods, she should replace high-sugar, high-fat foods with the nutrient-rich calories of eggs, lean meat, fish and poultry, low-fat milk and cheeses, whole grains and a lot of fruits and vegetables.

Does the nursing mother need the same amount of food or more or less than she required while pregnant?

She needs more food than she required during pregnancy. She is meeting all her previous responsibility—and taking care of a new baby, too. And she produces milk, often a quart or more a day, once nursing is established. She needs more protein, vitamins, calcium, and other minerals. In short, the same wholesome foods she ate during pregnancy, but more of all of

them.

Is breast milk still the food of choice for the newly born?

Yes, indeed. It always has been, and still is, their ideal food. Breast-fed babies get less sodium than those fed cow's milk, which may help them to avoid hypertension later in life. They also are less likely to become excessively fat. (Every baby should be encouraged to move about as much as possible.)

No child also eating solid foods needs more than a quart of milk a day. The new foods are richer in iron and copper, which are essential for forming red blood cells. If the child fills up on milk, anemia may result.

If you blend your own baby food, remember: prepare it fresh and keep it cold, for bacteriological safety. Don't salt or sugar it. The baby doesn't need it. It needs vitamin D and (if it isn't getting enough fruit juices) vitamin C.

Is it true that as the child gets to be eighteen months or two years old it seems to eat less?

Yes, for it is growing more slowly than it did during the earlier months. And it's eating adult food out of large dishes, which makes the quantity of food it consumes look less than it actually is. No matter what our age, good nutrition is a matter of what foods are eaten through the day, not at what hours. If a toddler prefers five meals, add a couple nutritious mid-morning and mid-afternoon snacks.

But don't make them sweets or desserts—and don't use such foods as bribes or rewards. The last thing you want to do for his teeth and his health in general is to condition him to think of sweet, empty-calorie food as something somehow superior to good, nourishing food. In fact, restrict all sugary foods and avoid high-fat foods as well.

Within reason, children are entitled to some preferences and dislikes. Your husband has his, you have yours. Just replace the abhorred food with something equally nutritious: meat by fish and eggs, one vegetable by another. And don't regard play activity as a form of self-indulgence. Encourage it as much as possible.

It used to be I was the only mother on the block who didn't bottle-feed. Now there seem to be several other nursing mothers around. Is breast-feeding really coming back?

I am happy to say it seems to be, at least among the more affluent and educated families. I wish women were getting more encouragement in this direction. At the White House Conference on Food, Nutrition and Health, a panel recommended that doctors and nurses do more to educate mothers in breast-feeding, and asked maternal health services to work for adequate diets for low-income nursing mothers. The panel said that, "All other things being equal, the mother who nurses her baby establishes, at an early date, an intimacy with her child which makes further relationships with him easy and natural."

The panel added that breast milk is the perfect food for a baby's nutritional needs and development and that it provides protection against infections and allergies that cannot be duplicated.

I'm breast-feeding my baby and my mother says I should drink a lot of milk. But I don't want to gain weight. What should I do?

Stop worrying, unless you're eating a great deal more of other things as well. In order to produce milk, your body can use up as many as 1,000 calories a day, particularly if your baby is a very good feeder. In fact, you're lucky. Most women who breast-feed get back to their pre-pregnancy weight much sooner than women who do not. Count all the calories, including those in the milk you're drinking each day. But subtract about 800 calories from your daily allowance to take into account the energy you use up lactating.

I am expecting a baby and want to breast-feed it. I am also a vegetarian. I am told that I need to drink milk in order to produce milk. Yet the biggest milk-producers in the world —goats, cows, female elephants and what-have-you—seem to manage perfectly well without eating animal products. Why should I be so different?

This question pops up with some regularity. Cows and goats (and some other animals) have four stomachs. One of the stomachs—called the rumen—contains enormous amounts of bacteria. These bacteria synthesize first-class, animal-like protein from hay or grass. These bacteria are digested in their turn.

You have only one stomach. And it does not harbor protein-synthesizing bacteria. Your baby will require calcium from your milk, in addition to protein, and you do not want this calcium to be drawn out of your bones. Unlike the cow, you never could eat enough vegetables to replace the calcium you need to secrete.

I am expecting my first child in a few weeks. I was planning to bottle-feed my baby. But after reading what you say in support of breast-feeding I've changed my mind. I've discussed it with my obstetrician, who doesn't seem interested, one way or the other, in how I feed the little one. Is there somewhere I can get some good information about breast-feeding?

Your first step should be a visit with your pediatrician. It's good practice, anyway, to meet with your baby's doctor sometime before your infant is born. You may find that he or she is quite enthusiastic about breast-feeding and able to provide you with all the information you need.

Unfortunately, however, too many physicians and too many hospital obstetrical departments are either disinterested or negatively disposed toward the nursing mother. The main reason for this hostility seems to be that bottle-feeding is easier for the nursing staff to administer: the mother—sleepy, sentimental and slow—is not involved, and the amount of milk taken by the child is clearly visible. The baby does not have to be moved from the nursery and away from the supervision of the head nurse. Yet, breast-feeding should be a simple, unintimidating method of giving an infant the best possible nutritional launching.

Most women can breast-feed successfully, and the process can be flexible enough to include even the working mother.

You may benefit, however, in the early weeks from having access to someone who can answer specific questions and provide on-the-spot reassurance.

Write to La Leche International, 9616 Minneapolis Avenue, Franklin Park, Ill., 60131, for the name of a representative near you.

I will be having my first child in about two months and am planning to breast-feed. One of my friends told me that chocolate is taboo for nursing mothers. Is this true and are there other foods I should avoid?

First, congratulations on your decision to breast-feed. To answer your question: eat as much as you like so long as it agrees with you. Chocolate is no exception.

Sometimes strong flavors, such as raw onion or garlic, will go into the milk (occasionally in cow's milk, you can detect those flavors, from pastures where wild onion and garlic were growing). Such flavors are not harmful to the baby, and he or she probably won't object. Of greater importance is to make sure your diet is adequate to meet the requirements of milk production.

Breast-feeding creates an increased demand for all nutrients, especially protein, calories, calcium and vitamins A and D.

A good, basic diet for a nursing mother should include about a quart of milk a day, with cheese and some ice cream as substitutes. (If you're using skim or other low-fat milks, choose a brand fortified with vitamins A and D.) You should also have two generous servings of meat, fish or poultry, three or more servings of fruit as well as a couple of vegetables and four servings of enriched bread or cereals. Including whole milk, this core diet adds up roughly to 2,000 calories.

The Recommended Dietary Allowance—the nationally recognized standard for nutrition needs—sets the caloric requirement for lactation at about 3,000. So you do have room for a goodie here or there. Studies done in England, however, suggest that 2,500 calories may be adequate. The difference really depends on the stage of nursing, its duration and the amount of milk secreted.

I have a two-month-old infant who is allergic to regular milk. My pediatrician has put her on soy milk. He's assured me the baby will do fine, but I'm still concerned. What is soy milk and is it comparable to regular milk?

Soy-based formulas have been used for many years to feed infants allergic to the protein in cow's milk. A meat-based formula, as well as the one made from the pure protein casein, are used for the same purpose. But soy milks (made from the edible seed of the soy plant) are, by far, the most popular

109

alternative for the cow's-milk–sensitive infant. While the older soy products have a characteristic soy taste and odor particularly unpleasant to the mother, newer forms made from isolated soy protein seem to be more palatable and produce fewer side effects. In addition to soy for protein, these formulas also contain oil as well as corn sugar or sucrose for adequate calories. They are fortified with additional nutrients.

Studies on infants fed soy-based formulas generally indicate that these babies grow quite as well as infants fed regular milk. So be reassured: your baby is getting adequate nutrition for his needs.

What is the modified food starch used in so many baby foods, and why is it used?

Modified food starch (MFS) includes a group of chemically altered natural starches used in strained and junior dinners, high-meat dinners, desserts and fruits. As used, MFS supplies between 10 percent and 32 percent of the calories available in these foods. This is high, but one survey of infant diets showed that this amounted to only a little over 2 percent of the total caloric intake for the day.

The starch is used to give the food a desirable texture and to keep the components of the product uniformly distributed, even under conditions of high speed manufacture. In practice, this means all foods with starch added have a similar, pudding-like consistency. Baby-food users have observed, for example, the difference in texture between applesauce made without MFS and plums containing starch. The applesauce is just a more finely puréed product than the adult variety, while the plum is indeed a pudding. The use of MFS in baby foods has been questioned.

The argument of baby-food companies is that their studies have shown that the use of natural starches shortens the shelf life of the product. They also say that much less MFS is needed to achieve the desired results than is required when natural starch is used.

A subcommittee of the National Research Council which reviewed the available information on modified starch found **110** that the risks of using MFS were nonexistent—or, at most, minimal. There was no reason, the researchers decided, to exclude MFS from infant diets, provided the standard now in existence be strictly enforced and that only the necessary amounts of starch to achieve a beneficial effect be used. On the other hand, the NRC subcommittee urged the FDA *not* to approve any additional uses of MFS until their safety has been demonstrated. They stated there was a lack of sufficient clinical evidence on the metabolism of MFS.

You can, of course, prepare your own baby foods, free of MFS as well as salt and sugar. Remember, however, that safety is essential. Prepare your food fresh and preferably don't store it. If you have to store it, do so in small containers so that you do not thaw it repeatedly.

> *My husband and I are both substantially overweight. We now have a six-month-old son and I'm determined to fight probability and keep him slim if at all possible. I use commercial baby foods and am wondering if there are significant differences in caloric content among the various fruits, vegetables and meats.*

First of all, if you haven't done so, you should express your concern about weight control to your pediatrician, who can tell you whether your child is indeed gaining weight too rapidly. If so, it is desirable to select baby foods with similar nutrient content but fewer calories—a "lower caloric density."

Caloric values for a given product can vary significantly from one manufacturer to another. The key factor is the amount of such things as sugar and modified food starch added by the manufacturer.

For example, applesauce with apricots: one brand contains 100 calories per jar, a second 120 and a third 130. Thirty calories isn't much for an adult, and a baby should probably not take more than a half a jar of fruit at meals, or only 15 extra calories for that portion. But remember that an average six-month-old baby requires only 750 calories a day, so that's 2 percent of them.

A second variable occurs within food groups. A half jar of carrots or squash from one manufacturer contains 17 calories, but a half jar of sweet potato contains 45. The difference of 28 calories represents almost another 4 percent of the day's energy needs.

This is clearly a case where calorie-content information on the label greatly aids the conscientious mother. Until such data are available for all foods, the only way you can know how many calories of a product you're serving to your child is to write to the manufacturers of the brands you use and ask them to send you the calorie information.

There are a large number of books on the subject of making your own baby food. One even mentions such exotic fare for an eight-month-old baby as Quiche Lorraine. Do you really think there's some benefit in going to the trouble of creating gourmet treats for such small children?

There is no great mystery about preparing baby food. It requires only a knowledge of the same principles of good nutrition, food handling and storage which apply to feeding adults. Add to that your pediatrician's specific advice about such things as the introduction of solid foods and the sizes of servings.

The idea of creating special dishes to excite little junior's palate seems a lot of work for very little return. Making your own baby food is time-consuming and not particularly economical if you're cooking especially for baby.

If you're simply using today's leftovers for baby's dinner tomorrow night, fine, so long as the foods contain the basic elements of good nutrition, are lightly salted or not salted at all, and were promptly refrigerated after cooking. If those leftovers happen to include cheese custard from Quiche Lorraine, that's okay, too. But I think that eight months is a bit premature to educate a youngster to the delights of classic French cuisine.

In general, remember that safety is the first commandment when dealing with baby foods.

If you make your own, don't keep it more than twenty-four hours in the refrigerator.

Don't freeze and thaw foods repeatedly.

Don't add sugar to baby foods. He or she doesn't need the empty calories.

Don't salt to taste. The baby doesn't need the salt and **112** probably doesn't taste it, anyway.

I put a lot of effort into preparing a meal that I think my two-year-old son will like. Sometimes he eats it. But sometimes he just makes a mess and eats virtually nothing. Why is this?

You imply you are cooking special foods for your son. By the age of two he should share the family fare. His appetite can be a whimsical thing. What he eats enthusiastically one day or even most days, he will reject another day for no apparent reason. It may be because he's tired, or had too many snacks close to mealtime, or he simply may not be hungry.

At lunch time try eggs, cold meat, sardines, fruit, milk—foods that require little preparation. That way, you've wasted only a small amount of food, not your energy, if he doesn't feel like eating lunch that day. If he rejects dinner, suggest a simple substitute. If he rejects that, forget about food until breakfast (unless he is really hungry later). Do not, however, offer dessert as a bribe. This will only lead you straight down the potentially dangerous path of using sweets as reward foods.

There are some questions you might ask yourself about your son's failure to eat well. Are you loading his plate too full? On an ordinary dinner plate, you may think (particularly if he's your first child) that the amount of food he requires looks meager. But it's better to give small servings and let him ask for seconds.

Are his between-meal snacks too large? A two-year-old has a small capacity. He probably can't take in all the food his body requires at three meals a day. If your doctor is satisfied with your child's growth and activity, your youngster is undoubtedly getting the food he needs. Put trust in what the great physiologist Walter Cannon called "the wisdom of the body."

I have a two-year-old daughter whose weight is already becoming a problem. She loves to eat and is always asking for a snack. Her father describes her size as "toddler, two, portly." What should I do?

There are a number of ways to prevent her cute chubbiness from turning into a life of obesity. First, find out why she's always asking for food. Is she really hungry or does she just want to get your attention?

Try to get her mind off her stomach. One easy way is to

do your kitchen work while she's napping. Just being around food and watching you cook it may give her the idea of eating. Otherwise, keep her occupied as much as you can.

Then, too, there are many ways to control the caloric content of a snack. Children can be just as happy with a dish of pickle slices or shredded lettuce as with a bag of potato chips. In fact, children really don't know about potato chips, candy and cookies as snack foods until we adults teach them.

You can even make the container more important than its contents. Children love their own personal bag of something. If you fill the bag with four plain crackers instead of three chocolate chip cookies, you've served approximately 60 calories rather than 150.

Another good do-it-yourself container is a small paper cup. Fill it with small pieces of apples and raisins or carrot sticks. You may also aim at establishing a regularity to feeding, such as three meals, two snacks and perhaps some juice at bedtime. Your child will get the idea that eating, like other pleasures, is only a sometime thing.

12 THE YOUNG

       If a child tends to plumpness or is downright fat, parents often lull themselves with the wishful thought that "he or she will grow out of it." But the evidence strongly indicates that many of today's overweight children—particularly girls—will probably be tomorrow's fat adults. Instead of growing out of their obesity, they grow along with it. And they are in grave danger of developing the outcast psychology that goes with feeling different.

       Surprisingly, most overweight children have moderate appetites. The problem is that they are abnormally inactive. Thus, in theory, the solution is simple. What the overweight child needs most is a regimen of moderate exercise, along with a diet low in sugar and fat. The diet is especially important in view of the recent evidence that cholesterol, associated with degenerative heart disease, often begins to lodge in the arteries during childhood.

Just what is an overweight child?

       Perhaps the best definition is that the child is carrying more *fat* than he should, a definition that puts the emphasis on fat rather than weight. Children, like adults, vary considerably in build, and it is difficult to determine the normal weight for a given height simply by referring to a statistical table. For example, two boys of the same age may be of the same height and weight, yet one of them could be too fat.

What is the chief cause of excess weight?

Heredity. Or, more precisely, heredity determines the *tendency* to overweight. This tendency is nurtured by a society in which food is plentiful, automobiles a way of life, and physical chores all but vanished from most households.

Studies reveal that the number of overweight children born to normal-weight parents in the United States is relatively low, averaging less than 7 percent. Yet, if one parent is overweight, the percentage rises to 40. And if both are overweight, their offspring will almost certainly be overweight too. The theory that environment, rather than genes, is the determining factor is refuted by evidence that children who were adopted at birth do not conform to these statistics.

If my child appears to be too fat, what do I do about it?

The first step is to consult a doctor. He'll know whether the extra weight is merely the puppy fat of pre-puberty, particularly if your child is in the eight to fourteen age group. Such a condition is often self-correcting. But if the weight is well over the normal before age eight and after age fourteen, it is likely to remain there unless the child gets some help.

The doctor will probably advise you to work on three key factors involved in taking off weight: (1) sound eating habits, (2) proper exercise, and (3) psychological support to curb possible emotional problems.

Most people believe fat children overstuff themselves at every opportunity. But many scientific studies reveal, surprisingly, that most overweight children not only have moderate appetites but often eat less than normal-weight children of the same age. Moreover, they do not consume any more sugar or fat than other children.

Then why does their diet have to be watched?

Because they are, as a rule, too lethargic to burn up what they eat. Therefore, the foods high in calories (but low in minerals, vitamins and protein) should be eliminated from the menu.

This means items such as sugar, candy, soda pop, high-fat dishes and especially rich cakes and pies which are high in both fats and sugars. It would be well, in fact, to keep these tempting items out of the house altogether.

Apart from these restrictions, however, the overweight child must get nutritious, well-balanced meals. It will certainly not help to put a child on a crash diet to lose weight. That could stunt growth, cause menstrual irregularity and create havoc with school performance and discipline.

A child should never be encouraged to skip meals, either. He can tolerate this kind of deprivation even less than an adult.

Once the caloric adjustment has been made in his diet, the crucial factor is exercise. With proper exercise, the child will eventually gain height, thus *growing into his weight.*

How was the importance of lack of exercise in the development of overweight in children established?

The first clue came out of a study made by a group of us at Harvard. Continuing observation of a number of obese Boston children revealed that they almost invariably gained weight during the fall and winter, their most inactive periods. A corollary study with adult male animals disclosed that when they exercised below a certain level they still continued to eat as much as ever and piled on weight.

Following these studies, we then compared the dietary and exercise habits of 56 high school girls, 28 overweight and 28 of normal weight. The overweight girls actually ate less than the normal girls, but were markedly less active.

Thereupon we tested overweight boys. They also had average appetites, coupled with extreme physical inactivity. Further studies by other researchers repeatedly confirmed our results. The findings were even true in research with babies. Fat babies were placid, and moderate eaters. Elongated and highly active (and highly vocal) babies ate considerably more.

To clinch the case, a four-year-long experiment with fat children showed that regular exercise did not boost appetite or food intake and, as a result, did slim them down. Thus all observations and tests conclusively proved that exercise, which may be defined as the expenditure of calories through body motion, is vital in preventing and treating overweight in childhood and adolescence.

How much exercise does an overweight child need?

At least an hour a day on weekdays and three hours a day on weekends. The type of exercise is unimportant. It's the intensity and continuity that count. But the greater variety of sports a youngster participates in, the more likely he is to find one that really delights him. It is hoped he can find at least one —such as tennis or swimming—he can continue to enjoy as an adult. If he does, he won't quit exercising—which happens all too often—as soon as his school days are over.

Though we have only limited data on the adult weights of overweight children, the most intensive study to date strongly indicates that fat youngsters generally grow up to be fat adults. Conducted in Maryland by Doctors S. Abraham and M. Nordsieck, the survey shows that over 80 percent of the extremely overweight boys and girls studied stayed that way as adults. Similar investigations in Western Europe have reached the same conclusions.

What can parents do to help their overweight children in their struggle with this problem?

They should try to join in their physical activity, even if this means only some brisk walking together. Parental participation often works wonders, for the parents as well as the children. Success in sports—no matter how modest—should be praised, since approval of the parents is as important as that of friends, sometimes even more so.

Girls, even more concerned about their appearance than boys, should be shown how to dress and do their hair to the best advantage, but only if the parent can do this with cheerful encouragement rather than with any implication of criticism.

Parents must be careful to avoid making derogatory comments about their child's appearance—even in jest—since the overweight youngster usually has a low opinion of his or her body and personality and is easily depressed. In addition, parents should take every opportunity to reassure the child that he or she is loved and esteemed.

118

What other problems does the overweight child have to face?

Like adults, the overweight youngster is under constant pressure to reduce. He or she is belabored by radio, television and magazines as well as by family, friends and classmates. He or she is made—because of this experience—to feel like an outcast.

While the overweight child may have the same IQ and school grades and be no more guilty of absenteeism than the normal weight child, he or she nevertheless often has great difficulty in getting into the college of his or her choice—or even into college at all. Discrimination is particularly savage against fat girls. With equal grades, overweight girls have only one-third as much chance of being accepted at top eastern colleges as do girls of normal weight, overweight boys two-thirds as much.

Little wonder then that overweight youngsters typically show psychological traits of heightened sensitivity, preoccupation with self-image, passivity, and expectation of rejection. All these, in turn, make the child more isolated and less active. A self-perpetuating cycle develops. The time to correct the situation is before it has a chance to develop into a lifelong handicap.

My small children ate lunch at a friend's house the other day, and the mother served some new product being marketed "for children who won't eat vegetables." It looked and tasted quite like french fried potatoes. The ingredient description listed potatoes first, then powdered peas and powdered carrots. Is this really a good way to get children started on vegetables?

While her motives are excellent, this mother may in effect be reinforcing her children's fondness for french fried potatoes.

Vegetables are liked less by the junior set than are most other foods. And it's unreasonable to expect every child to like all vegetables. While we hope they will eventually broaden their taste horizons to like most of them, the best plan is to go slowly. Serve youngsters' favorite vegetables like carrot sticks, green pepper rings and tomato wedges (all quite high in vitamins and minerals). Add a small amount of those they like less and make sure that they eat a variety of fruit (orange juice, though excellent, is not enough).

Above all, don't make an issue over a refusal to eat vegetables. Nutritional health does not hang on a stalk of broccoli.

Our community is divided on school lunches. A school committee says only cold school lunches can be provided this fall. But an active group of concerned parents maintains cold school lunches are nutritionally inadequate and that children require hot lunches. Is that true?

From a purely nutritional viewpoint, a cold lunch can be adequate. What determines the nutritional value is nutrient content. And a cold meal can contain just as many calories, just as much protein, just as much of the essential nutrients as a hot meal. And if the meal is well conceived, it can be perfectly well digested.

A meal, however, should provide more than nutrition alone. A good school lunch should be a moment of rest and relaxation, a time for pleasant companionship and for conversation with classmates and perhaps with teachers under other than classroom conditions.

Atmosphere is important. The room should not be too crowded, it should be pleasantly decorated and it should not be too noisy.

My children are forever nagging me to take them to one of the hamburger drive-ins that seem to be on every second corner nowadays. I'm wondering just how much meat they're getting in these hamburgers.

As you might have guessed, you'd better not count on that hamburger as your children's major source of protein for the day. The standard cooked hamburger contains an average of slightly over one ounce of ground meat. In order to keep prices down, some chains are beginning to add small amounts of textured vegetable protein as extenders. Even so, the cost of a hamburger on a bun is twice what it would be if you served the same thing at home, using plain ground beef containing 30 percent fat, the legal limit for fat in hamburger.

When it comes to drive-in food, hamburger on a roll and **120** plain milk are probably the best nutritional offerings. The rest of the menu is generally devoid of vegetables (except french fried potatoes) and fruits (except in well-sugared pies) and heavy in high-caloric sweet drinks.

While it would be foolish to hope that the ubiquitous hamburger stand will quietly go away, try to keep them on your list of "for special occasion" treats and not the place the family eats every other day.

> *I'm a teen-ager. And to me hamburgers and french fries are the greatest. But my mother is always knocking them. She says they aren't as good as real meat and vegetables. Please tell her she's wrong.*

I'm one of the nutritionists who don't knock hamburgers and french fries. There's nothing wrong with them as such. In moderation, they're not going to harm a young person who's active. Indeed, they are high in calories. So they are not for dieters. And they—especially those you get at roadside stands —are high in fat. Obviously they're not the sort of food for an adult male, whose cholesterol is rising, to live on.

Otherwise, I'm all for them. The important thing is to eat enough fruit and vegetables and drink milk at other times of the day.

(P.S.: Mom, there's nothing to be gained by being puritanical about food. Just make sure that over the course of the day the overall food intake of your child is adequate, however bizarre and possibly unbalanced some of the individual meals may be.)

> *Surely (a mother asks) you do not mean teen-agers could live on such a diet?*

Indeed, I do not. All I mean is that, as part of a balanced diet, hamburgers and french fries are not bad foods for a physically active youngster. They certainly do not constitute a complete diet. Active youngsters need a sufficient amount of vegetables and fruits to get their complement of vitamins and trace minerals. They need milk or skim milk or yogurt or cheese to get enough calcium. They need salad with corn oil, peanut, cottonseed or safflower oil to improve the ratio of polyunsaturated to saturated fats.

The quality of their diet will be further improved if you

choose as lean a grade of ground beef as possible and grill the
hamburger, letting the fat drip out. Fry the potatoes under
cover in corn, peanut or safflower oil. I hope they will also eat
fish and poultry each once or twice a week.

*By now everyone must know that carrot and celery sticks,
dill pickles, and assorted other greenery are tops on the list
of nibble foods for dieters. But, frankly, this just isn't exciting enough for my teen-age daughter. She's a bit plump but
certainly in no need of a starvation diet. What can you
suggest?*

First, more exercise!

But what you're really asking for are some snack-food
suggestions. So-called rabbit food certainly can get a bit dull
after a while. But, since you say your daughter has no need for
strict dieting, there are many snack ideas which range in the
under-200-calorie category.

A cup of unbuttered popcorn, for example, has about 55
calories. Six three-ring pretzels have 72 calories. A small bowl
of dry cereal with skim milk, 110 calories; add half a small
banana to it for a total of 150 calories. A half of a peanut butter
sandwich, 165 calories; pizza made with half an English muffin,
American cheese and a tomato slice, 180 calories. A piece of
fruit is always a good idea at about 50 to 80 calories, depending
on the type of fruit and the size of the piece.

But, remember, if she's going to eat up calories in the form
of snacks, there has to be a corresponding sacrifice at mealtimes. Or the inevitable unhappy result: more calories are consumed than are burned, and more weight is gained.

What are the nutritional merits of junior dinners?

There really is no particular merit in using them instead
of regular canned foods. As with infant foods, there are two
types of junior foods. First are the regular junior dinner or
junior vegetables-with-meat. These supply relatively little protein, with most of the calories coming from starch. Second are
the junior high-meat dinners, which cost more and supply
nearly twice as much protein. Calories for the two products are
roughly the same.

122

A combination of junior meat and junior vegetables provides the most protein. And it teaches the child to appreciate individual food taste and colors. Unfortunately, the available number of plain junior vegetables is limited. And too many are marketed in cream sauce, cream sauce with bacon, or butter sauce, which add mostly calories.

Once a youngster has graduated from children's food, the time has come to start thinking beyond baby products and increasing the use of the food the rest of the family eats. The cost difference is significant. For example, compare the cost of a jar of junior spaghetti with tomato sauce and beef with the price of a can of spaghetti in tomato sauce with cheese you heat up for the rest of the family. You'll find that the junior food costs twice as much!

What can you do about children who never want to eat regular meals but are starving for snacks when they get home from school?

Give them submarine (hero) sandwiches. It's one of the best snacks because it has a little bit of everything in it. Not so easy to eat, maybe, but it's good food. A cookie, a glass of milk, and a piece of fresh fruit are nutritious, too, but I prefer a sandwich. Peanut butter is particularly good; it's high in polyunsaturated fat and protein.

My son and daughter, aged eight and ten, are both on the heavy side. Can you suggest some after-school snacks for them?

Since snacks for children must be considered in the context of the day's total food intake, the amount of calories allowed is somewhat variable.

Your children may prefer simply to redistribute their calories, and eat only half a sandwich at lunch, saving the other half until after school.

If they are fortunate enough to go to a school where there is a choice of items available at noon, they can be encouraged to select lower-calorie dishes in order to be able to have a larger afternoon snack.

In some homes, where dinner is delayed until late so the family can eat together, a substantial afternoon snack may be quite necessary. In order to avoid weight gain, calories must be borrowed from other meals, and this requires planning.

Fruits rank among the most nutritious low-calorie snacks. Encourage children with weight problems to eat a piece of fruit rather than take a glass of juice. Juices, of course, are perfectly good, but children can quickly consume substantial quantities. (A medium apple contains 70 calories, but a cup of apple juice has 120.) A cup of vegetable soup containing 80 calories is another good idea. Or try a slice of American cheese and two saltines, at about 100 calories.

By avoiding such things as cake, potato chips and other obviously concentrated sources of calories, it's possible to provide a snack of greater volume with fewer calories.

I am a high school student. My interest in nutrition has been stimulated to the point that I'd like to learn more about the field and the career opportunities it offers.

You might start by watching some nutritionists and dietitians at work in your community. You'll find them in hospitals, in neighborhood health centers, in the Extension Service, in school food service, and in the state and local health departments.

Also, you might explore state universities that have programs in nutrition and dietetics.

The American Dietetic Association, 620 N. Michigan Avenue, Chicago, Ill., will provide you with printed material and refer you to a nutritionist or dietitian in your community with whom you can explore career opportunities more fully.

I pack my children's lunchboxes early in the morning and they don't eat lunch until four or five hours later. I've heard that mayonnaise can spoil if it's not kept cold. So should I stop giving the children their favorite tuna fish sandwiches?

It is the *combination* of mayonnaise with tuna—or, for that matter, other fish or meat—that creates a breeding ground for bacteria unless the food is kept cold. These organisms upset the stomach if the food is not consumed a few hours after it's made, particularly if the temperature is high. On hot days, you may want to give the children something else in their lunchboxes. But serve the tuna fish for dinner or on weekends; it's a great way to get them in the habit of liking fish.

Our local church runs a morning nursery school. We are thinking of expanding to a full day-care program and hope to serve snacks and lunch to the children. Are there federal funds available, and how does one find out about them?

Yes, indeed, there are funds available for child-feeding programs other than those in public schools. These funds are administered by the Food and Nutrition Service of the Department of Agriculture. The money, allocated by Congress, may be used for day-care centers, day camps, and summer recreation programs. It is unfortunate that in past years some of the money allocated for this purpose has not been used simply because no one has asked for it.

To find out whether your organization is eligible, contact the director of school food services at your state department of education.

Remember, many of the problems involved in planning nutritious and appealing meals for groups of children on a regular basis are quite different from those encountered in feeding one toddler in your own kitchen.

You'll probably find that you can use some help. Check with the people at the school food service department to see what nutrition personnel and materials are available from their organization to help you get started. They will also know of resources at the local level on which you can call. You may be pleasantly surprised to find that help is available for the asking.

I've read about a spongy, cupcake-like product, equal in nutritional value to an egg, two pieces of bacon, four ounces of orange juice, a pat of butter and a slice of bread. The article which introduced it to me criticized the idea of feeding children a sweet piece of cake in the morning. How do you feel about this?

The idea of having food available to all school children, rich or poor, in the morning is a good one. Far too many children come to school with nothing in their stomachs. In fact, there are many children who plainly cannot get breakfast down when they first arise in the morning. But they are ravenously hungry by the time they get to school. (How many adults **25** operate this way, too?)

Some schools do serve a breakfast of fruit or juice and cereal with milk. Others are unwilling to get into the food business early in the morning. It is especially in these schools that a nutritious product like the one you describe has a place. It is, indeed, high in sugar, and this is a serious drawback, from the dental viewpoint in particular. But it is a first step in developing a complete meal in a single package. We hope that very soon nonsugary convenience breakfasts will be available in the schools, more sandwich-like than cake-like.

> *Our grandson is allergic to eggs and milk. We are at a loss to put some variety into his meals. Can you recommend some sources of allergy recipes?*

Here are three specific suggestions:

The American Dietetic Association's "Allergy Recipes," available from the A.D.A., 620 N. Michigan Avenue, Chicago, Ill., 60611, for $1.00.

"Baking for People With Food Allergies," from the Superintendent of Documents, U.S. Government Printing Office, Washington, D.C. 20402, for 10¢.

Good Housekeeping's "125 Great Recipes for Allergy Diets," from Goodhousekeeping Bulletin Service, 959 Eighth Avenue, New York, N. Y. 10019, for 50¢.

Many commercial food companies have free nonallergic recipes. The nutrition section of your state health department can supply you with their names and may have some allergy recipes of their own.

> *My two teen-agers drive me out of my mind with their irregular food habits. First, they don't like some of the foods that everybody else eats. They refuse eggs and bacon at breakfast. One wants a cheeseburger. The other is on a wheat-germ kick. Then, instead of eating lunch and dinner, they snack all day long. What can I do to make sure that they are well fed?*

A cheeseburger is a very good source of protein and calcium. Wheat germ is a low-fat source of protein, B vitamins and vitamin E. If it is consumed with milk, it is a good source of protein, vitamin B_2 and, again, calcium. Make sure that they have some fresh oranges, orange or another fruit juice (not a soft drink) high in vitamin C, and they can be on their way.

As for the rest of the day, it would be nice if they could have one organized meal—say, dinner—both because it does give them a balanced meal and because it provides a good opportunity for conversation.

Try to avoid buying snack foods high in fat, high in salt, often made from unenriched flour, which contribute mostly empty calories.

Stack up on whole-wheat or enriched bread because they are high in B vitamins and iron. Whole wheat is a source of trace minerals and vitamin E. It is also a good source of roughage, useful in avoiding constipation, and perhaps in preventing diseases of the large bowel in later life. Buy also low-fat milk with nonfat milk solids added.

Tunafish, sliced ham or cheeses, may be moderately expensive, but they are excellent sources of protein. Have plenty of fruits and nuts of various kinds around the house. Again, nuts are good sources of protein as well as of polyunsaturated fats. If you can teach your teen-agers to concoct elaborate salads with a variety of ingredients, you won't have to worry about their nutrition.

Is breakfast a more important meal for children than it is for other members of the family?

It is, indeed. Children's metabolism is faster (they use up their food more rapidly) than that of grownups. Unless young people start off the day with a good-sized, balanced meal, long before noon rolls around they might be operating without adequate reserves. They may not be as alert as they need to be and their learning may be impaired.

I've become headmaster of a small boarding school for boys and was surprised to find that chocolate milk is available in unlimited amounts at both lunch and dinner and is consumed in great quantities. Should I banish the beverage?

Perhaps as a long-range goal you will want to explore the idea of developing a program of nutrition education to help the boys make their own appropriate decisions about food selection.

As for chocolate milk, it is hard to condone the use of

unlimited sweets at meals, but cutting them out completely is probably a rather drastic step. Just as you might do for your own son at home, put a reasonable limit on chocolate milk—say, no more than one glass per meal, or make it available at only one meal a day, perhaps supper.

The prepared chocolate milk sometimes available is made of skim or partially skimmed—not whole—milk. It is flavored with chocolate, and may have added stabilizers which give it that viscous consistency. It may or may not be fortified with vitamins A and D. One cup contains roughly 190 calories, about 30 more than the same amount of whole milk and more than twice as many as a glass of skim milk. But in many parts of the country chocolate milk is not available. The usual product is "chocolate drink" or "chocolate flavored drink." Often it is completely synthetic, except for water.

Two groups of youngsters, in particular, should be discouraged from drinking chocolate milk. Obviously, an overweight boy should be encouraged to opt for the lower-calorie milk. And the youngster whose appetite is poor should also be steered away, at least until the end of the meal. Sweets tend to temporarily depress the appetite. The boy who is already a poor eater may drink the chocolate milk and leave much of his balanced meal untouched.

We have in our schools vending machines offering a substantial amount of what I consider junk food. I'm afraid that too many of the children patronize them rather than eat the school lunch. How do you suggest combating this?

The vending machines need not be there forever. You might solicit support from other mothers and fathers who feel as you do and, as a group, speak with the school administration about your concern. Ask a local dietitian or public health nutritionist to help organize your presentation and have your nutrition facts in order.

Then there's the child-centered approach. Your youngsters are exposed to all types of food in all kinds of situations besides the school situations where they are clearly the persons making the choice. Many factors influence their decisions. It is estimated that the average child is exposed to no less than 5,000 food-related television commercials a year which can have a significant effect on his choices. There are also daily after-school snacks on the way home which too often include a soft drink and some sort of cake.

Much of the solution to combating all this lies in education. Schools, and particularly, school food services, are putting increasing emphasis on this area, and this is good. There is no reason, however, that the responsibility for educating children in proper food selection cannot begin at home. This can be done both through logical explanations and by the example of the type of food brought into the home.

But begin early. Even an eight-year-old child can be taught about the harmful effects of sugar on the teeth.

13 THE AGED

To be old anywhere is difficult. And in many ways it is more difficult in the United States than in many other Western countries. This nation has never been kind to the aged. It was settled by young people who left their parents behind, first in English cottages, later in German cities, Irish farms, eastern European ghettoes, Sicilian villages and Norwegian fishing harbors.

Today, promotion and job transfers keep younger people moving while the elderly stay put because they are "too old to travel" or they "wouldn't want to leave friends behind." They are often too old to keep house for themselves, too poor to keep up repairs on their homes and have anything left over. Their friends who are their contemporaries are also disinclined to go and visit unless they are transported door to door and helped in and out of the car.

All of this has a real effect on their eating habits and nutrition. The elderly are handicapped in many ways. Their financial resources are meager and can be reduced drastically by even one lengthy stay in the hospital. To outward appearances many may be living well, but they could be starving in comfortable surroundings simply because maintaining those surroundings requires so much of their income. Many old couples might well be eligible for food stamps, but would rather die than apply for them at the welfare office. Indeed, some literally do die.

The elderly also may be nutritionally handicapped by arthritis or poor vision, both of which inhibit them from doing the shopping, opening certain kinds of packages, and preparing and serving food. Lack of teeth may keep them from eating comfortably.

Living alone, they are disinclined to spend much time or effort cooking and are discouraged by the inconvenient sizes of many processed items. All in all, the elderly tend to subsist on soft foods such as buns, pastry, cereals and baby foods—not only a monotonous diet but one often low in essential nutrients.

All this means that you *cannot* take the good nutrition of your elderly relatives for granted. They may seem to be eating well when you visit them by invitation. But try dropping in unexpectedly, when they haven't prepared a show for you.

At the risk of appearing to have lost your manners, ask questions about the kinds of food they regularly eat during a week. Get specific. Check the cupboards and refrigerator for an idea of what's going on when you're not around.

If you have an elderly relative in a nursing home you should be aware that some of these institutions all too often attempt to save money on food, to the point where the meals are not just unpalatable but do not meet basic needs.

What are the basic food needs of the elderly?

First of all, they require food for energy. This need tends to decrease with age, but probably not as much as many think. It declines rapidly between the ages of forty-five and sixty-five, but relatively slowly from then until the age of seventy-five, when it stabilizes. Inactivity is an additional question. Men and women in their sixties or seventies need about one-third fewer calories than they did in their twenties. If they continue to exercise moderately, however, they may need more.

Do older people often make mistakes of judgment in selecting particular foods?

They do. Because they are often afflicted with chronic diseases about which medical science can do little, they are favorite targets for quacks who urge them to squander their precious food dollars on "miracle foods" instead of spending them on the variety of nutritious, everyday items they require.

What the aged must be made aware of, before all else, is that while their overall need for food may well be less, they need to get more food value per amount of food. The concentration of nutrients—proteins, vitamins and minerals—should be a matter of primary concern.

If, on the advice of a physician, the older person takes a supplement, it should be one with all the vitamins at the Recommended Dietary Allowances level, and containing the recommended—or estimated—allowances of minerals, particularly iron. "Megadoses" of single vitamins or minerals are expensive, useless, sometimes dangerous and should be avoided.

Is osteoporosis more common in older men and women?

Osteoporosis, usually associated with the aging process, is the loss of minerals, particularly calcium, from the bones, causing a gradual decrease in total bone tissue. The bones are brittle and break easily. Many physicians prescribe fluoride, calcium and vitamin D supplements. Calcium can readily be obtained from milk and cottage cheese, which are also sources of protein. The elderly should pay more attention than young people to reduction of saturated fat, salt and sugar. Fortunately, when fat and sugar are cut down, they are usually replaced by foods higher in vitamins and trace minerals.(See Chapters 5 and 6.)

Is alcoholism frequently encountered among older people?

It is all too common among the elderly who live alone, and many too often drink more than they should. This drinking will often be associated with eating less frequently and less wisely than one should, thus further compromising good nutrition.

What about laxatives?

Well, another problem compounding poor nutrition is the use of brutal laxatives such as mineral oil, which drain away vitamin A and other fat-soluble vitamins. Occasionally, a mild laxative may be useful, but continued need should be brought to your physician's attention. Far better

132 than laxatives would be the inclusion in your daily diet of several servings of fresh fruit as well as a cereal high in fiber, such as bran.

Are the elderly more menaced by undernutrition than they are by overnutrition?

While undernutrition is the more common problem, over-nutrition is equally a danger to the elderly. People often think that there isn't sufficient reason to put an old person on a reducing diet and that it is even cruel to take away the pleasures of the table from one who is so old anyway. It would be good to remember that overweight itself takes away many of the joys of life and interferes with such fundamentals as walking and self-care. Injured and weakened bones may not be able to stand an additional twenty or thirty pounds. It is no favor to the old to let them eat as much as they like. The alternative to a diet may be the nursing home or worse. At the same time, crash diets, a threat at any age, may be especially harmful to the elderly.

I'm a senior citizen and my physician told me to eat one cup of oatmeal seasoned with margarine every night because I was about ten pounds underweight. It really is working. What is it about oatmeal that's particularly helpful in gaining weight?

Absolutely nothing. But if you've kept your eating and exercise habits fairly constant and added a cup of cooked oatmeal with about a tablespoon of margarine, you've added about 250 calories a day. Since it takes 3,500 calories to make a pound, in a month's time, you should have gained a little over two pounds.

At that rate, in less than five months, you'll get out of the featherweight class. Just remember that's when to call it quits on your daily food supplement.

The strength of the remedy is that you've been given a very specific assignment that you've followed. Incredibly enough, that's all it takes to make it work. I receive considerable mail reflecting concern about being on the lighter side.

First of all, if you're otherwise healthy and have always been thin, it probably shouldn't be of serious concern. But for **133** those of you who think you'd feel better with a few more pounds, the device of adding a daily snack without changing anything else about your eating and exercising habits can be effective.

> *On a recent visit to an old aunt who's living alone, I discovered that her diet consisted largely of baby food. Can baby food provide adequate nutrition for an adult over a long period of time?*

Yes. A reasonably nutritious, though not terribly appealing diet can be provided using baby food if the proper ones are selected and eaten in adequate amounts.

For example, a lunch consisting of a jar of junior meat, a jar of junior vegetables, and a jar of fruit for dessert, served with a slice of bread and butter or margarine and a glass of milk, would provide more than a third of the day's nutritional requirements.

If, however, lunch is a vegetable-and-meat combination, with some fruit and a cup of tea, the diet will be lacking in several nutrients, including protein, as well as in calories.

Nutritional adequacy is important. However, one must be concerned about the reason your aunt has chosen to eat baby food. Is it poor-fitting dentures? A lack of interest in eating? Is it that she just doesn't feel like cooking for one person? Does she have some digestive distress that needs to be evaluated by a doctor? Surely it can't be because baby food provides a tremendous taste thrill.

Many elderly people resort to baby food or a diet of milk and crackers simply because they've lost interest in the whole business of cooking and eating. If you find there's no real problem other than boredom, you may be able to find help in your community. One alternative for your aunt might be eating some of her meals with other people of her generation. Some senior citizen agencies offer low-cost, nutritious lunches or dinners.

> *I've heard somewhere about home-delivered meals for older people who have difficulty getting out of the house to shop. What are these programs and how can I find out more about them?*

The services to which you refer are generally called Meals-on-Wheels. Usually they are run by one or more voluntary agencies who deliver a hot meal to elderly people in their homes. They also often serve meals on a communal basis (in school cafeterias, in the evening, for example).

You might call your local Visiting Nurse Association or public health department to find out if there is such a service in your community and, if there is, how it operates.

> *I have an aged relative in a nursing home. Am I right in assuming that he is being provided with plenty of good food containing all the nutrients he needs?*

Unfortunately you may not be. Nursing homes run all the way from the excellent to the appalling. Some of them are everything you'd want them to be in the meal department. Others are not.

Ask the opinion of observant physicians who visit patients in the particular home where your relative is staying. Politely ask a few of his more alert fellow guests. Visit the home, without previously announcing your impending arrival, at mealtimes. Sample some of the food yourself.

14 SAVING YOUR HEART

I am constantly reminded of the kill-joy image nutritionists are acquiring. Not too long ago, a nutritionist was pictured as a rather jolly, middle-aged lady who went around the countryside preaching a message of more milk, fruit, vegetables, meat, fish, whole-wheat bread, butter, cheese, eggs and—again and forever—more milk.

She was not terribly popular, but everybody appreciated her. Grandmother had known the truth all along. Mother used the nutrition-lady's argument to force additional food on her unwilling children. Of course, she was applauded by the farmer, the food industry, the U.S. Department of Agriculture, and the legislatures of the farm states.

Alas, times have changed. Today the nutritionist is a hostile, male fanatic whose chief passion is to snatch away from you all the good, "rich" foods of this land of milk and honey. His message is downright un-American: fewer calories and less sitting.

Both recommendations go very much against the grain of a country that spends billions to advertise a greater and greater number of convenience foods, a country whose whole economy rests on the manufacture of every conceivable labor-saving device, and whose national pastimes are to sit at home watching television and to sit in large stadiums observing a handful of paid professionals exercising in their behalf.

The nutritionist preaches less fat, less butter, less hydrogenated vegetable fat, less *whole* milk, certainly less fat meat. And here we are with a whole system of meat grading based on marbleized meat, made tender by the infiltration of fat in the muscle of the beef cattle through the use of every nutritional and hormonal technique available!

The nutrition expert preaches less cholesterol, in a country where the ghost of Theodore Roosevelt still seems to be proclaiming, "Good men eat breakfast." Everybody knows he meant two fried eggs and plenty of bacon and buttered toast.

The nutritionist preaches fewer sweets in a country where "sugar" is a standard term of affection.

Furthermore, the admonitions seem so unnecessary. After all, your grandfather ate the good things you are being warned against, never counted calories, had two eggs and bacon every morning, ate meat every time he felt like it, put sugar in his coffee, and lived to be over eighty.

What is so new that we have to change all these pleasant habits? Isn't this new attitude just one more manifestation of our national puritanical streak which at various times has prohibited the theater, the dance, the demon gin, tobacco, and now, in a more chemically oriented society, is against dietary calories, sugar, fatty acids, and cholesterol?

Unfortunately the new attitude cannot be dismissed that easily. The fact is that something *new* has happened, and so catastrophically that nutritionists have felt they had to embark on a midnight ride to wake a slumbering countryside. The new factor is the explosion of coronary heart disease, so sudden in terms of generations and so widespread that it can only be called "a new epidemic."

It may seem almost incredible that it is only in the twentieth century (and well into the lifetime of your grandfather) that coronary heart disease and myocardial infarction—the final closing of a narrowed coronary artery—became adequately described. To be sure, the student of the history of medicine, exercising hindsight, could find vague descriptions of

137

chest pains in the medical literature of the ancient Egyptians and Greeks. He would find also that the great English anatomist Harvey did perform, in 1647, an autopsy on a middle-aged man who had "distressing pain in the chest" and had died during one such episode. But we must jump to 1912 before a classification of coronary obstructions was published in the United States.

And in the 1918 medical publication that first reported the changes in the electrocardiogram during a myocardial infarction, coronary disease was said to be "so uncommon that most medical students and house officers never heard of the disease during their period of clinical training." It was only in 1944 that the electrocardiograph in its present form—so familiar to any middle-aged man who has had a thorough checkup or insurance examination—came into use.

Finally, it was as late as the 1950s that routine determination of blood cholesterol was started and in the '60s that attention was given to other blood fats.

What are the signs and symptoms of a coronary?

In a typical episode they are usually so dramatic—severe chest pressure and pain, nausea and vomiting, ashen pallor, cold sweat, clammy skin, rapid and feeble pulse, pain in the left arm, low-grade fever, blood changes and fall in blood pressure —that we must give credence to older physicians' universal recollection that the disease was indeed exceptional in the first part of this century.

Just how extensive are coronary attacks?

This disease accounts for nearly half of the deaths of males over age forty in the United States. A condition that only the most erudite specialists could have identified as recently as 1930 is so common now that it can be diagnosed by the average person.

This drastic development—paralleled only by the arrival of bubonic plague in fourteenth-century Europe, syphilis from the New World at the end of the fifteenth century and pulmonary tuberculosis at the beginning of the nineteenth century— explains the profound change in attitude of nutritionists, cardiologists and other health professionals. Nutritionists display what may seem to be an almost fanatical anxiety toward dietary habits because they know we are faced with an emergency. If unchecked, the situation could statistically cancel the effect of this century's entire progress in medical knowledge and medical care.

What changes have brought about this almost unbelievable increase in heart disease?

First and foremost, our mode of life has shifted. In the late 1890s, physiologists classified the normal activities of man as "sedentary," "moderately active," "active" and "very active." The terms are still in use today. But what a difference of definition has occurred!

In 1895 a "sedentary" man was typically a clerk. He got up at 5:30 A.M., split wood or shoveled coal for an hour to stoke the family fire, walked an hour to get to the office, spent ten hours at a stand-up desk, walked back home, and spent another hour with ax, hatchet or shovel to prepare for the night. On Sunday (his only day off) he once again worked to keep the home fires burning, walked his family to church, and then took everybody walking in the public park or the countryside, played outdoor games, or took care of his garden.

A "moderately active" man was a factory worker who put in long hours from the age of fourteen on, doing hard jobs without benefit of modern labor-saving devices.

An "active" man was a plowman or carpenter working his tools.

A "very active" man was a ditch-digger, a lumberjack or a miner who spent up to sixty hours a week with his ax, pick or shovel.

There were no automobiles, telephones, school buses, washing machines, cotton-picking machinery or bulldozers.

But doesn't our participation in sports provide us with sufficient activity to replace that previously provided by farm and factory?

Most adults do not take part in sports at all, and the activity over long periods of most of those who do is negligible. Most sports-oriented grownups today are spectators. Indeed, the last remaining body motions, however trivial, are being

139

eliminated; the manual shift of your automobile has been replaced by automatic gears, the manual typewriter by an electric. The installation of one more telephone extension eliminates a few more steps. All this has brought a degree of immobilization that was unknown even to the wealthiest citizens of America and western Europe in past centuries.

Hasn't the body changed to adjust to the lessened demands made on it?

The human body is still the same! It was developed through millions of years of evolution to run, fight and work hard. Studies in my laboratory have shown that the appetite mechanism of even normal persons which under more natural conditions equalizes food intake and energy output is often unable to function at these incredibly low levels of activity. You eat more than you expend, like caged or cooped up animals, and inexorably you become fat.

Not only that, but lack of exercise is also accompanied by a tendency to increased blood pressure and decreased elasticity of the blood vessels. Overweight among children has increased. Coronaries are no longer exclusively a disease of old age, but also of men in their forties, their thirties, even their twenties.

All this has happened in the course of a few decades and is the high price we pay for a civilization in which we have used technology not just to eliminate back-breaking work, but to eliminate—from kindergarten through retirement—almost all physical effort.

Is the extreme cutting down of demanding physical effort the only change in the pattern of our lives that makes us more vulnerable than previous generations to the danger of heart disease?

There have been other such changes. Cigarette smoking, rare in men and unknown in women in 1900, has become the rule rather than the exception for both sexes.

The diet, meanwhile, has correspondingly evolved from one high in bread and potatoes to one rich in fat and cholesterol (eggs, whole milk, meat) and sugar. Even in families whose diets have changed least, the mode of life that made such a diet tolerable has changed.

How early in life does the prospect of heart disease become a matter of concern?

Much earlier than we suspected. We have been used to thinking of atherosclerosis as a disease of the middle-aged and elderly—because that is when we see, particularly in men, the well-known signs of the disease: coronaries, strokes, angina, and the diseases of the kidneys, the eyes, ears, hands and feet that result from damage to the arteries.

But, during the Korean War, three U.S. Army physicians performed 300 autopsies on American war casualties and examined their coronary arteries. In over three-quarters of the cases, gross coronary artery disease was present in these men whose average age was only twenty-two years. Other studies showed no such damage in Korean soldiers, killed alongside them.

During the Vietnamese War, another team of U.S. Army doctors once again found widespread coronary damage in the hearts of very young Americans killed in action. A large study examining the state of the heart in a number of countries again showed atherosclerosis (hardening of and damage to arteries through production of cholesterol-containing deposits) to be much more common in young men in the United States than in most other areas of the world.

If our young men already showed such damaged hearts when they barely reached adulthood, does it mean that the precautions against heart disease currently advocated are being taken much too late?

Yes, in fact a considerable amount of existing evidence indicates that a high-fat diet can push the cholesterol level of even a thirteen- or fourteen-year-old dangerously upward. Yet this increase can be readily controlled. A few years ago my colleagues, Drs. McGandy and Stare at Harvard's Department of Nutrition made limited changes in the students' diets at two nearby prep schools and were able to cut by nearly 50 percent the rise in blood cholesterol that usually takes place between fourteen and eighteen.

Just how "limited" were the changes in meal-content made at these schools?

All eggs were eliminated in one school except for once a week and in the other except for twice. They were replaced by a low-cholesterol substitute. Polyunsaturated margarines were used instead of butter. Students were served more fish and poultry. Pork and beef remained a part of the diet, but were carefully trimmed of fat. For desserts the researchers concocted a special low-fat ice cream. I was sufficiently impressed to suggest to the University Committee on dining halls that such changes be applied at Harvard, and found that our academic administrators are indeed becoming interested in cardiovascular prevention.

Are successful attempts to lower the blood cholesterol of teen-agers enough to guard against arteriosclerosis?

No. Lowering blood cholesterol is an important measure, but there are other major steps that should be taken. Hypertension is the other major risk factor in heart disease. Lewis K. Dahl of the Brookhaven National Laboratory found very significant correlation between sodium intake and blood pressure. Approximately 65 percent of sodium consumed by the average American comes from convenience foods. Careful policing of labels for data on salt content can be a protective step.

In addition, the effects of overweight on the young are extremely disturbing. All existing studies indicate that onset in childhood definitely contributes to a shorter life span. And lack of exercise in the young is another material risk factor affecting an increasing number of young people. The effect of overweight and high blood pressure combined is worse than either one alone and constitutes a real and present danger. If a child is overweight and its blood pressure is up, she or he should try to bring her or his blood pressure down by increased exercise and decreased intake of calories and salt.

I come of a long-lived family. Doesn't that increase the chances that I, too, will live a long life?

All of us have to stop leaning on the fact that Grandfather lived to be a very ancient man. Granted, there is still a statistical advantage in familial longevity. But the way your grandfather lived, particularly when he was still young, was so different from the way you and, even more, your children live that he is an unsuitable example for you to follow.

If you want to live in good health as long as Grandfather did, you will have to do several things Grandfather did *not* do. First of all, you must take steps to decrease the fat content of your diet to no more than a third of your total calories. A good start is to cut down on ice cream, butter, pastry, and fat meats, and to use skim milk. At the same time you should increase the ratio of polyunsaturated to saturated fats. You should also adjust your carbohydrate intake so that you eat fewer foods containing sugar. Your diet must be planned to avoid—or reduce—overweight. And it's wise to reduce the amount of salt you eat to ward off high blood pressure.

If you are still a smoker, try your very best to stop completely. At the very least switch from cigarettes to a pipe or cigars.

Since you are not going to work as strenuously as Grandfather did, you must exercise. If you're already out of condition, begin slowly to get back in shape. As a sort of insurance, have a complete physical, particularly if you are going to plunge into a fitness program.

If you're in pretty good physical shape, stay in top form by paying attention to your living habits. If you have to give up or reduce some energy-using activity, find a substitute, and make sure it uses up about the same amount of calories. If it doesn't, cut calories.

What specific effect does exercise—or the absence of it— have on the development of heart disease, aside from controlling weight?

Although it has by no means been conclusively proved, it's possible that exercise may delay the development of hardening of the arteries. What is fairly well established so far is that exercise stimulates the growth of new sources of blood supply to the heart even during the development of artery disease.

This was shown clearly in laboratory experiments with two groups of dogs. First, the main artery to the heart was constricted (narrowed) in each animal by tying a ligature around it, and then the animals were divided into two groups.

One group exercised on a treadmill, while the other group had no such activity. When the animals were examined, all of them had developed additional (or what scientists call "collat-

143

eral") blood vessels to make up for the restricted flow caused by the narrowed artery. But the additional circulation was much greater among the exercised dogs, and in some of them the collateral network was so developed that completely normal circulation had been restored to the heart.

What conclusions might be drawn from this experiment with the dogs?

It would suggest that during the early stages of general hardening of the arteries (which takes place as we grow older) exercise might be particularly helpful.

Since most middle-aged American men probably have an early, invisible degree of narrowing of the arteries, it seems imperative to encourage those who have no sign of heart trouble to get busy exercising. Even those who have had a recent coronary attack might benefit by exercise, so long as it is not strenuous enough to cause pain.

A cardiologist, a specialist in cardiac rehabilitation, is the best judge of how much exercise is appropriate.

Does the nature of the exercises you do for the health of your heart matter very much?

The nature of the relatively intense exercises you do is really of little importance, provided a large enough fraction of the total muscle mass is involved. The larger the muscle mass, the greater the heart response. Exercise which involves the legs and the back muscles is thus preferable to exercise which is performed primarily by the arms.

Push-ups essentially involve the muscles of the arms and shoulders, whereas running, rowing, and swimming involve most larger muscles. While it is desirable for a younger man still in good condition to exercise an hour daily, with an expenditure of 700 calories, the simple fact is that three fifteen-minute periods of intense exercise a week, together with a daily hour of walking, are sufficient to improve cardiovascular fitness to a considerable extent.

Of all the recommendations you make for us to avoid heart disease, which is the simplest?

It is true some recommendations are more difficult to carry out than others. It is a complex task to modify your diet. You may feel it's impossible to give up smoking. It's not always easy for you to get plenty of exercise. And losing weight is notoriously difficult. But one vital thing you can do for the health of your heart is simplicity itself. Take the salt shaker off the dinner table. And cut down on salt in cooking.

Of all the factors which predispose so many people to these conditions, which is probably the most dangerous?

Hypertension—high blood pressure—is one of the chief predisposing causes of heart disease, because it makes blood vessels of the heart, kidneys, brain and eyes much more susceptible to atherosclerosis, or "hardening" of the blood vessels due to accumulation of calcium and cholesterol in their walls.

Loss of mental capacity, and senility, because of poor transfer of oxygen, glucose, and other nutrients to the brain, are all too frequent effects of atherosclerosis.

Worse still, high blood pressure is the overwhelmingly dominant risk factor in the development of strokes. Prevention of high blood pressure—which affects upward of 10 million Americans—thus emerges as one of the most important aspects of health maintenance.

The single most vital step in detection of hypertension is a yearly physical examination. When high blood pressure has been diagnosed, medication is usually prescribed. It is generally the single most important factor in the treatment, but reducing the salt intake, weight loss and regular exercise are also highly useful and often give powerful aid to drug treatment.

What does all this have to do with taking the "salt shaker off the dinner table"?

A universal prescription for hypertension is cutting down on the salt intake, which may mean marked or even drastic reduction. Since the main goal of drug treatment of hypertension is to eliminate as much sodium as possible from the body, cutting down salt in the diet obviously helps control hypertension.

Cutting down salt in the diet appears also to be a factor in prevention of high blood pressure. Dr. Lewis K. Dahl of the Medical Center at Brookhaven National Laboratory divided a large number of adults into three groups, depending on how much sodium they consumed.

He found that over 10 percent of the group with high intakes of sodium had hypertension, compared with 7 percent of the average group, and less than 1 percent of the low group. Conversely, in another study, hypertensive subjects were found to have a higher salt intake than those with normal blood pressure.

Breast milk has a very low sodium content, a concentration lower than that of tap water in many cities. Cow's milk is much higher, over three times the concentration in breast milk. Dr. Dahl found that when thirty varieties of baby foods (all of which showed a sodium content greatly in excess of that of the unprocessed meats and vegetables from which they were made) were fed to baby rats of a strain predisposed to hypertension, high blood pressure developed within four months. In the past few years there has been a tendency for some manufacturers to cut down on the salt in baby foods, but there is still too much of it in U.S. foods. (The Swedes have eliminated salt from their baby foods altogether.)

Are other age groups also exposed to the risk of oversalted foods?

Mothers, themselves conditioned to a high-salt diet, unnecessarily add salt to the eggs and other dishes of small children. Children and adolescents are increasingly exposed to the temptations of snack foods, which, when they are not extremely high in sugar, tend to be extremely high in salt.

The trend continues in adulthood, when many Americans automatically pour generous amounts of salt out of the shaker before they have even tasted the food—which has, as often as not, been well salted before it was served.

Many of the packaged convenience foods are very high in salt. Some canned soups, excellent though they are otherwise in terms of nutrition, are also very salty. And restaurants often give you little choice but to eat highly salted dishes.

Are you suggesting we eliminate all salt from our cooking?

Not unless told to do so by a physician. What I am suggesting is that we cut down on the amount of salt we use and substitute for it what has always been the basis of tasty cooking, the careful use of bay leaves, thyme, sage, marjoram and other herbs, and lemons, onions, peppercorns, black and red pepper, paprika, horseradish or mustard seed and, for those who like it, a touch of garlic or garlic powder. Use wine vinegar and fine-flavored oils.

Then you're not out really to take the fun out of food?

To the contrary. The more appetizing you can make the food you serve, the better off everyone is. There are some foods that can be almost magically transformed by just a pinch of salt. But just a pinch. A month hence, once you are used to the new level of saltiness, your food will taste as salty as it does now. Remember that the main reason large amounts of salt used to be necessary is that brine kept bacteria from growing in foods that our ancestors did not know how to can or freeze and couldn't refrigerate. With modern methods of food preservation, we can remove this unnecessary hazard from our environment and with it the peril brought by excess salt.

I've often read about arteriosclerosis and atherosclerosis. Do both words mean the same thing?

Arteriosclerosis is a general term, including almost any arterial disease which leads to thickening and hardening of the arteries.

Atherosclerosis is a specific form of arteriosclerosis. Fat accumulates on the inside walls of certain arteries of the body. The progressive development of atherosclerosis is the main cause of coronary heart disease, stroke, and gangrene of the extremities.

My doctor advised me to cut down on cholesterol. If I use unsaturated margarine most of the time and my wife cooks with unsaturated oil, can't I have a little butter now and then? Can I also use mayonnaise?

The idea is to reduce the *total* amount of fat you eat and to shift from foods containing saturated fat to foods with unsaturated fat. It would be foolish, in fact impossible, to eliminate all saturated fat. But these two steps—cutting down on total fat and substituting polyunsaturated fats for saturated fats whenever possible—are vital factors in the fight to lower blood cholesterol.

Of course, you can have some butter and mayonnaise. But, remember, avoid meat fat and whole milk or cream as much as possible, and cut way down on eggs.

When the picnic and cook-out season comes around, my husband is a great participant in these affairs. But his cholesterol is high. Is he better off eating hot dogs or hamburgers?

I am sure your husband's physician would agree that neither of these two foods could be a staple in a cholesterol-lowering diet. But as long as your husband limits the number of his hot dogs, he is better off with them than with the hamburgers. A hot dog contains about half the calories—and half the amount of fat—of a hamburger. Why don't you take along cold chicken to your picnics?

I am a middle-aged man with an average cholesterol level —240 I think the doctor said. He advised me to go easy on breakfast eggs and I have cut down from two eggs every morning to two a week. But my neighbors tell me that they have heard that soft-boiled eggs don't raise your cholesterol because they contain lecithin. Is this true?

Unfortunately no. I know the lecithin myth is going around; it was perpetuated by a popular writer on the basis of her misunderstanding of the biochemistry of cholesterol in tissue, which does involve lecithin. Lecithin aside, the fact is that you can raise a person's blood cholesterol by adding eggs, which have a large amount of cholesterol, to his diet—particularly if the diet is otherwise low in cholesterol. One famous study proving this fact was conducted by my colleague Dr. D. Mark Hegsted in the Nutrition Department of the Harvard School of Public Health. With his associates he found that, in adult men, the average level of blood cholesterol goes up 5 milligrams for every 100 milligrams of cholesterol eaten daily in the diet. Two eggs contain 500 mg. of cholesterol; the corresponding increase in blood cholesterol was 25 mg. per 100 milliliters. Dr. Ancel Keys, another well-known researcher, has found an even greater effect in his studies, adding cholesterol to a low-cholesterol diet. He believes the rise would not be quite so dramatic if the diet were already high in cholesterol. Keys also found that polyunsaturated fat in the diet tended to somewhat reduce the jump in blood cholesterol when cholesterol was fed.

I am a man in my mid-thirties. Recently, I learned that my blood cholesterol was very high. Through a new program of exercise and a diet high in polyunsaturates, I've managed to reduce my cholesterol count considerably. My problems arise in eating out. So many items on a restaurant menu are taboo that there is no choice. Do you have any suggestions?

Among the smartest places you could eat is an Oriental restaurant. Usually the fat used for sautéeing is liquid oil. And there is a large variety of fish, shellfish and chicken dishes. Avoid the few deep-fried dishes on the menu.

Food selection, even on a cholesterol-lowering diet, is not an either/or question. Some foods, while not highest in polyunsaturates and lowest in cholesterol, are far better than others. In an Italian restaurant, for example, you'd be better off with spaghetti and clam sauce than spaghetti and sausage.

Menus in American-style restaurants offer some options. Unfortunately most Americans still look forward to the juicy steak. Where fish is available, it remains the best choice. And it is not unreasonable to have your order broiled or cooked in oil rather than butter.

Roast chicken is a better choice than fried. In any case, avoid eating the skin. Veal roast is leaner than rib roast of beef. A tomato sauce is likely to be lower in fat than a cream sauce. While your choice is limited, there are options. If you eat out frequently, you'll do well to choose restaurants that offer enough options.

I know that cheese is considered high in both fat and cholesterol, but I'm wondering if some cheeses contain less than others?

Cheese does contain considerable fat and cholesterol but there is a wide variability among the different types of cheeses. In general, as the fat content rises, so does the cholesterol, though this is not a hard and fast rule.

Researchers at the Agricultural Experimental Station at Rutgers University undertook a chemical analysis of some thirty varieties of cheese, domestic and imported. It comes as no surprise that cottage cheese is lowest in fat and cholesterol. Then comes farmer cheese and mozzarella, followed by Danish samsoe, French brie, Muenster, American and Italian Bel Paese.

Cheddar, a popular cheese in this country, is quite high in fat, but contains less cholesterol than blue cheese and Roquefort, which were measured the highest.

Do egg noodles really contain much egg? And, if so, are they a serious consideration as part of one's cholesterol intake for the day?

Egg noodles do contain egg, but probably not enough to be of concern unless you're eating quite a large amount of them every day. An 8-ounce box of dried noodles would still not contain as much cholesterol as one egg. And that's a lot of noodles.

In more practical terms, a cup of cooked noodles made with whole egg contains about 50 milligrams of cholesterol, or about a fifth as much as is found in an egg. A word of caution: small amounts of egg used in cooking and in mixed food can quickly add up to an egg a day or more.

I've been reading about a study which found that people who drink a lot of coffee have more heart attacks than do those who don't. Will you tell me more about this?

One indictment of the beverage made from the coffee bean comes from some rather controversial data collected by the Boston Collaborative Drug Surveillance Program.

Researchers found, through questioning hospital patients who had a coronary and those who had been admitted for other conditions, that men and women who drink more than four cups of coffee a day were twice as likely to have a heart attack as were those who abstained from it.

While there was a correlation between coffee drinking and cigarette smoking, the reason for the relationship between coffee drinking and heart attacks remains a mystery.

One theory is that heavy coffee drinkers are striving, competitive, "coronary-prone" types. Or it may be that there is an unknown substance in coffee that makes heavy consumers more susceptible to heart attacks. Both caffeine and sugar have been

150

ruled out. Some tea drinkers consume similar amounts of both but no substantial correlation between tea drinking and heart attacks has been found.

It may be added that prospective studies, in which people are followed through yearly checkups and diseases or causes of death are recorded, have not shown any striking correlation between coffee drinking and coronaries. Obviously, more research is needed to clarify the possible relationship, if any, between coffee drinking and coronaries.

In the meantime, what is the coffee drinker to do? The answer, I think, is moderation. Coffee drinking can become excessive—up to ten or fifteen cups a day. And if all that coffee contains cream and sugar, the caloric intake can be substantial. It is not unreasonable to set five cups as an upper limit.

15 OTHER MEDICAL MATTERS

Sometimes it appears we are rapidly becoming a nation of "nutritionites."

A nutritionite—it is my own word—is not a nutritionist. A nutritionist knows he has limitations. He is aware that some areas of the body of knowledge called nutrition are firmly established, others less so. Gaps still wait to be filled.

The nutritionite is less knowledgeable and less humble. Out of his own ignorance, his misunderstandings of fragments of nutritional commonplaces, and his delusions of omniscience, he sounds off, he directs, he advises.

Nowhere is he more conspicuous than in the field of sickness and the care and feeding of its victims. The most dangerous nutritionites are sick people who—with the best will in the world, the will to be well—practice nutrition of sorts on themselves.

I am gratified that among the hundreds of letters that reach me each week so many come from ill people who are neither nutritionites nor victims thereof. Among the following questions from my mail are many heartening examples of the latter:

I have hypertension. And I'm on a 1,000-calorie-a-day diet and take drugs my doctor has prescribed. Am I going to have to stay on this diet for the rest of my life?

I assume that the reason for the 1,000-calorie diet is that you need to shed some weight. Weight loss often has a dramatic effect on the control of hypertension. A 1,000-calorie diet, as I'm sure you have already found out, is pretty restricted.

Your doctor is probably aiming to reduce your weight fairly rapidly to a reasonable level. Once you have achieved that goal you must be careful about your food intake lest the pounds you've fought to lose creep insidiously back.

For the average, moderately active adult, a 1,000-calorie diet need not be a life sentence but more or less a quick means to an important end.

The chief of pediatrics at a large medical center said that he hoped that within twenty years humans would, after weaning, stop drinking milk. He said that there were possible hazards of excess fat from whole milk, that milk drinking caused anemia, and that lactose intolerance is more common than we think. I suspect he is overstating the case, but can you set me straight?

You're quite right. It is overstated. It is true that some children consume large quantities of milk, which is poor in iron, to the exclusion of virtually all other food. These children gain weight and can, in fact, be chubby, though anemic. This type of iron-deficiency anemia is easily preventable, if mothers are counseled about the importance of introducing iron-rich foods, like baby cereal, and advised about the hazards of excess milk drinking.

Lactose intolerance, or the inability to handle milk sugar, is currently a subject of great interest and debate. While a substantial number of people, particularly nonwhites, may be lactose intolerant, the extent of the intolerance varies. Many can still tolerate some milk without unpleasant gastrointestinal effects. Lactose intolerance is far rarer in infants than in adults.

The emphasis on a diet lower in fat and cholesterol makes good sense. To that end, skim milk, fortified by vitamins A and D, is certainly a wise choice for adults. And it can certainly be

153

used for at least part of children's milk intake, especially where a weight problem exists.

In these days of unprecedented concern over the food dollar, nonfat dry milk is probably the biggest bargain on the supermarket shelf.

I have a severe allergy to milk and milk products, including cheese. I'm concerned about whether I'm getting enough calcium in my diet. Are there any other foods high in calcium, or should I resort to dietary supplements?

With a diet completely lacking in milk and milk products, meeting the day's calcium requirement is a formidable task. Two cups of milk (skim milk contains as much calcium as whole milk) or two ounces of cheese are generally recommended as essential to a well-balanced diet to meet the major percentage of the day's calcium requirement.

A few other foods are quite high in calcium. Canned sardines and canned salmon, where the fish is eaten bones and all, are two. But one is unlikely to eat six ounces of sardines (that's about two cans) or nine ounces of salmon regularly enough to approach the body's need for calcium.

A cup of brazil nuts will supply about as much calcium as a glass of milk and a cup of almonds somewhat more, but most people aren't in the habit of eating nuts by the cupful on a daily basis. This represents formidable amounts of calories as well.

Other fairly good sources of calcium include: dried beans, green leafy vegetables, broccoli, oranges and green beans. But none of these are consumed in large enough quantities to make a serious dent in calcium needs. While it is possible to dedicate oneself to obtaining adequate calcium on a milk-free diet, it's probably not worth the effort.

This is one time when a dietary supplement is advisable. Before starting on calcium pills, however, check with your doctor about prescribed dosage. It is wise not to exceed the Recommended Dietary Allowance of 800 mg. a day. Massive doses can cause problems in some individuals.

I have an allergy to milk. Not long ago, I read something about "filled" and "imitation" milk. What are these products and can I use them on a milk-free diet?

Generally, no. Filled milk generally falls into two types. One is a combination of fluid skim milk, with or without skim-milk solids and vegetable fat. The other contains water, nonfat dry milk, vegetable fat and some additional protein such as sodium caseinate or soy protein.

Imitation milks usually contain such ingredients as water, corn syrup solids, sugar, a vegetable fat and some protein, such as sodium caseinate or soy protein.

In either case, a product containing sodium caseinate will provoke the same allergic response as milk. And both filled and imitation milks usually contain as their primary source of fat coconut oil, which is highly saturated.

Is there any connection between the consumption of sugar and diabetes?

There may be. A responsible Israeli investigator, Dr. Aharon Cohen, found that the Jewish refugees who came to Israel when it became a state (1948) or at the time of the Six-Day War (1967) from areas where sugar was unavailable (such as the Yemen) had essentially no diabetes. After a quarter-century of life in Israel, with plenty of sugar available, the proportion of diabetes among the 1948 Yemen refugees and their descendants has risen to the normal 3 to 5 percent (depending on the cut-off point in defining diabetes).

Doctor Cohen has further shown that rats selected for several generations for diabetic tendencies did not become diabetic on a high-starch diet but became so on a high-sugar diet.

We conclude that not only is sugar a forbidden food if you are diabetic, it is also one you and your children should avoid if you have a diabetic ancestry.

Would it be a good idea for people who, as far as they know, have no sugar-connected problems to cut out all sugar from their diets?

I wouldn't go that far. I would, however, encourage them to eliminate highly sugared cereals and to consume, instead, nonsugared cereals lightly sweetened with a small amount of sugar which they dispensed themselves.

I would say to any of them: sugar your grapefruit very lightly. Avoid eating any sugar at lunch or during the day when you cannot brush your teeth immediately thereafter. At the evening meal, eat fresh fruit for dessert whenever possible. Fruit canned in fruit juice should be your first choice. Light syrup is preferred to heavy syrup. Serve pies, ice creams, and cake only as special treats and brush your teeth or at least rinse well right afterward. You may not eliminate your consumption of sugar; but please try to reduce it.

Can sorbitol and mannitol, included in many dietetic products, be used by diabetics?

Sorbitol and mannitol, chemically, are alcohols which have been widely used as sweeteners. The former is made commercially from the simple sugar glucose, the latter from an ocean-growing plant, sea-tangle. Both occur naturally in fruits and vegetables, though sorbitol is more plentiful. In large amounts, both produce an undesirable laxative effect.

Both are absorbed more slowly than sugar into the bloodstream. From that standpoint, they would seem desirable for use in a diabetic diet. (Mannitol, in fact, is only partially absorbed.) But once absorbed, both are converted back to simple sugars. At the same time, they do contribute calories.

Most adults who develop diabetes in later years also develop a weight problem. Achieving a reasonable weight and holding it is one of the most important factors in the control of diabetes. Overcoming a sweet tooth is a difficult task, but it is unquestionably a better alternative than sorbitol-sweetened cookies. Remember that in addition to sorbitol, the cookies contain flour, eggs, shortening and other ingredients, all of which contain calories.

I am a diabetic and use lemon to season my food. My sister says that lemons have a lot of sugar. Is this true?

Lemons, like all other fruits, do contain fructose or fruit sugar. If you were making lemonade, using as much as a half cup of lemon juice with an artificial sweetener at one time, you would be getting about 40 calories, ordinarily referred to in a diabetic diet as one fruit exchange or one serving of fruit. But for using lemon juice as a seasoning on salad or fish, you needn't worry about the few extra calories you might consume.

How well established is the link between sugar and dental caries?

The relationship between sugar and tooth decay is one of the oldest and most solid observations in dental medicine. In the fourth century B.C. Aristotle asked, "Why do figs which are soft and sweet damage the teeth?" He did not know it, but figs are one of the rare fruits high in sucrose. And all modern studies have confirmed the existence of the link.

Populations which are not exposed to sugar, such as the isolated inhabitants of Tristan da Cunha and Yemenite Jewish immigrants in Israel, have been found to be essentially free from dental caries. So are families suffering from the disease "fructosuria" who avoid sugar carefully because it makes them sick.

Sticky forms of sugar, such as soft candy and chewing gum, appear to be the most cariogenic.

Is there any truth to the charges that sugar is responsible for both heart disease and cancer?

For many years Dr. John Yudkin, Professor of Nutrition at the University of London, has maintained that sugar, not saturated fats, was the main agent in the rise of blood cholesterol and heart disease over the course of the last century. Most nutritionists do not agree with this view.

There appears to be a small group of individuals whose cholesterol and serum fats are particularly sensitive to carbohydrates, but the majority of nondiabetic individuals are not in that category. Sugar is not implicated specifically in the development of cancer of the large bowel.

The evidence suggests that diets low in fiber (high in meat, milk, eggs, refined flour and sugar) promote diverticulitis and malignancies of the colon and rectum. It has been proposed that increasing the consumption of salads and certain fruits and vegetables (apples, raw carrots and the like) and, particularly, of bran cereals and whole-grain bread may be the answer. Certainly the other foods, such as refined cereals and sugar, would have to be decreased proportionately. But this is a long way from saying "sugar causes cancer."

I have diverticulitis and my doctor told me to avoid fruits and vegetables. Can you explain what diverticulitis is and what its relation is to diet?

Diverticula are outpouchings which can develop in weak spots in the bowel wall. When many of these outpouchings are present and one or more become inflamed—often causing pain on the lower left side—the condition is known as diverticulitis.

Virtually nonexistent in the early twentieth century, diverticulitis has been called a deficiency disease of Western Civilization. Its incidence has grown steadily in industrialized countries until between one-third and one-half the population over forty in the United States, Great Britain, France and Australia suffer from it.

Having ruled out hereditary factors, many physicians believe that diet is the culprit—that diverticulitis is a result of the increased use of refined flour and cereal and the substitution of foods containing large amounts of sugar and of meat for fibrous fruits and vegetables. In countries where the diet is high in residue and has changed little (among the South African Bantus or the Chinese, for example) diverticular disease is still almost nonexistent.

Logically, if the low-residue diet causes diverticulitis, the practice of using this diet for long-term management is questionable. In fact, an increasing number of physicians feel that a high-residue diet is appropriate. In Great Britain one group of researchers has had remarkable success in alleviating symptoms by simply adding bran to the diet.

I have suffered from severe psoriasis for a number of years. I go to a dermatologist and obtain limited relief from drugs. I've just heard about a turkey diet successfully used to treat psoriasis. Will you tell me something about this?

The concept that a low-protein diet might be beneficial in the treatment of psoriasis has been around for nearly sixty years. Studies with patients whose psoriasis has been resistant to drug therapy suggest that a low-protein diet may, indeed, have a positive effect. The turkey diet simply uses turkey as the major source of protein.

Originally, it was thought this regimen was low in tryptophan, one of the essential amino acids, and that the beneficial effects were due to tryptophan deprivation. This idea has been disproven.

It was also suggested that improvements observed on the turkey diet might be due to some special substance peculiar to turkey. This idea, too, has been discarded.

It is more likely that the substitution of turkey for other protein sources which may contain factors harmful to the individual with psoriasis is what produces the improvement.

Let me caution you, however, that the effectiveness of the turkey diet, as well as other dietary approaches to the treatment of psoriasis, is very much an open question. Before you lay in a stock of turkeys, discuss the appropriateness of trying something like the turkey diet with your dermatologist.

I have heard that the amino acid histidine is sometimes given for arthritis. Is this true and, if so, how much should I take?

Histidine is an amino acid known to be necessary for normal growth and maintenance in infants. It appears not to be one of the amino acids necessary for adequate nutrition in adults.

Not long ago, however, some investigators reopened that question. A report on the effectiveness of histidine in treating a group of rheumatoid-arthritis patients appeared in the literature: oral doses seemed to improve the arthritic's hand-grip strength and walking speed. But this method of treatment is still very much in the research stage. Discuss this with your physician.

Is there any nutritional advice you can give me that would moderate the extreme discomfort of arthritis?

As far as we now know, none of the rheumatic diseases is caused by a deficiency or an excess of any particular nutrient. The patient's diet should be varied and he should not become or remain overweight.

There is no evidence that too much calcium in the diet is the cause of the bony malformations that occur in osteoarthritis. An attempt to correct them by cutting down calcium intake may bring about osteoporosis, subjecting the sufferer to the possibility of serious bone injuries.

There is no justification for subjecting rheumatoid-arthritis patients to a diet of "sulfur-containing" foods or to an orange juice and cod-liver oil regimen. Listen to your physician and follow his instructions.

I have been taking the "Pill" for a few years. Recently, a friend told me she'd read that women who use oral contraceptives should take extra vitamins. Is this true?

A substantial amount of research has been done on the relationship between nutrition and the "pill." But few hard facts have been established and much uncertainty still surrounds the mechanism of the pill.

One undesirable side effect has been headaches, and there is evidence suggesting that the use of pyridoxine (vitamin B_6) will eliminate them. Exactly why this happens is still under investigation.

But before you rush off to the pharmacy to stock up on vitamin pills, I strongly urge you to discuss this further with your doctor.

I am in my middle sixties. Up until about a year ago I had rarely experienced any bowel trouble. But since then I frequently find myself uncomfortably constipated. What should I do?

Any distinct change in bowel habits, such as constipation, that lasts longer than a week or two, should be reported to your physician. You may then be advised about the proper fiber and roughage content of your diet, or further medical investigation may be undertaken.

I'm supposed to be on a bland diet for an ulcer that I developed a few months ago. Recently I started cheating and noticed that it didn't bother me. How long should I stay on my ulcer diet?

That is a question only your physician can answer. The American Dietetic Association published a statement about dietary treatment of ulcers which might, however, be of interest to you and your physician.

Three points are of particular significance:

First, studies that compare the effect of eating a bland diet with eating any diet you might choose yourself show that eating a bland diet made no significant difference in the healing of the ulcer.

Second, the weight of scientific evidence indicates that small, frequent feedings are helpful.

Third, intolerance to specific foods varies from patient to patient, which underscores the need for an individualized dietary plan.

In other words, the foods you have chosen to cheat on may not have caused you discomfort in the first place.

I've been told that the United States Army has developed a process whereby food is irradiated, and that this destroys bacteria, insects and worms. Will this really do such things? And is this process dangerous in any way? Could it cause cancer?

Several organizations, of which the U.S. Army is one, have discovered a remarkable method of irradiating food which can, apparently, perform wonders. It can kill bacteria in frozen meat without raising the temperature a degree, kill insects in a sealed container, and put an end to larvae, worms and molds. All this, of course, makes for the better preservation of food.

Irradiation, while of much promise everywhere, could be a blessing in such famine-prone countries as India, where each year up to a third of all harvested food is ruined by such intruders before it reaches the intended consumers.

Some irradiated foods have already been approved for human consumption by different governments.

Although early reports linking these foods to the appearance of cancer have been disproved, I am still cautious about the process and insist that irradiated foods be tested just as thoroughly as new additives are tested.

Does irradiation produce in food new substances about which we know nothing? Let's hope not. But let's find out!

I have a hiatus hernia, and my doctor says I should take antacids, not overeat, and avoid lying down after meals. What is hiatus hernia? Is there anything else I can do to help the heartburn I have as a result of it?

A hiatus hernia is a condition in which a portion of the stomach is pushed up through the diaphragm. Belching, pain in the lower chest and hiccuping after meals are, in addition to heartburn, common. These symptoms are the result of the contents of the stomach washing up into the esophagus and causing an inflammation there.

Hiatus hernias are quite common, although there are differences of opinion about their frequency. Estimates range from 10 percent to as high as 60 percent of the population. Fortunately, most hiatus hernias are asymptomatic; only a few cause sufficient illness to require medical attention.

Sometimes a bland diet with small, frequent feedings relieves the symptoms. As you go on your regimen, continue to check with your physician to see if further treatment is needed.

Is there a diet that is helpful in treating acne?

Unfortunately the role of food in the cause and treatment of acne vulgaris, or common acne, has traditionally been overemphasized. Enthusiasm for food restriction is currently less popular than it was.

Formerly, shellfish and iodized salt were often eliminated because it was thought that iodine had an influence on acne. This is now disputed. Chocolate is often regarded as bringing on acne, although one recent study found no evidence. If you personally find that a particular food, such as chocolate, causes flare-ups, avoid it.

But in general, the answer for most acne sufferers is first to have your skin problem evaluated by a dermatologist and, second, to be patient. In time, most acne just disappears. Above all, don't let anyone convince you that some fad diet will rid your skin of acne. It won't.

I recently was diagnosed as having gallstones and put on a low-fat diet. But I'm having trouble learning which convenience foods and snack foods are right for me. Can you tell me about fish sticks, frozen french fries and corn chips?

It is difficult to be specific in making suggestions, since individual tolerances vary. But there are a few facts which may help you. People with gall-bladder disease generally can best tolerate dairy fat (in limited amounts). The types of fat used in

162

the manufacture of the foods you mention are usually vegetable oils, and these are not digested as easily. Further, the amounts of fat these foods contain can vary considerably.

Fish sticks or frozen french fries are generally "blanched," or cooked for a short time in deep fat. As a result, four fish sticks may contain about the same amount of fat as a comparable serving of one of the fattier fish such as salmon, mackerel or pompano. While I might support the use of fish sticks as a meat substitute for someone on a cholesterol-lowering diet, individuals with gallstones might not tolerate it well.

Ten pieces of frozen french fried potatoes, if prepared in the oven without adding fat, contain about one teaspoon of vegetable oil. Mashed potato, made with only milk, might be a better selection, and is certainly lower in fat.

Snack foods such as corn chips, those popular powerhouses of calories, generally do contain considerable fat and are probably best left alone. If you can afford snack calories (that is, if they do not push up your daily caloric allowance) pretzels or unbuttered popcorn are wiser choices—but they may be high in salt.

Do you have a diet for gout I could follow, or a list of foods to eat or to avoid?

The dispensing of a particular diet for gout, or for any other condition requiring dietary management, must be left to your own physician, who knows the details of your case. But here are a few general comments about diet and gout:

Since early times, a relationship between food, drink and gout has been observed. Historically, doctors have used all sorts of bizarre dietary approaches to treat it. About a hundred years ago, the high uric acid levels in the blood of gouty patients were recognized. This served as a basis for what was the first rational dietary approach: a diet low in substances which form uric acid, a "low-purine" diet.

However, it has since been found that even in normal people only half the purines come from dietary sources. The rest are made from simple compounds readily available in the body. Thus the strict low-purine diet is no panacea, either.

Certain foods very high in purine, which is the immediate

precursor of uric acid, are usually restricted. These include sweetbreads, anchovies, sardines, liver, kidneys and meat extracts—foods generally sacrificed without hardship.

A number of authorities have noted that high-fat intakes decrease excretion of urates. On the basis of this evidence, some physicians prescribe low-fat diets.

However, one recommendation appears to have universal acceptance: if you have gout and you're overweight, reduce.

Not long ago I had a kidney stone removed. The doctor didn't put me on any special diet but advised me to drink a large volume of fluids. I'm wondering if there is any dietary measure I can take to prevent a recurrence.

Probably the most important measure you can take is to follow your doctor's advice. Other dietary measures are generally not considered practical for a number of reasons.

First, the substances from which stones are formed usually come in greater amounts from the body's metabolism than from outside food sources.

Second, since stones are made from a mixture of substances, dietary restrictions would obviously be impractical.

Finally, there really has never been any good evidence that dietary restrictions are effective in preventing kidney stones. Occasionally, when excess calcium is found in the urine, a low-calcium diet is prescribed. Other restrictions, based upon findings of abnormally high urinary levels of another particular substance, may also be useful. But such specific measures are rarely taken and then only after careful laboratory determinations have been made by a physician.

For several years, I have been afflicted—thank heaven, only after long intervals—with extremely troublesome migraine headaches. Could this be due to something in my diet?

Because many investigators feel food can play a part in causing attacks, migraine is sometimes classified as an allergic disorder. Among the foods most commonly implicated in precipitating migraines are chocolate, alcohol, dairy products and citrus fruits.

Monosodium glutamate, the flavor enhancer, has been
164 shown to cause "Chinese restaurant syndrome" in which head-

ache may be a prominent feature. Then there's something called "hot dog headache" which afflicts some people after they have eaten frankfurts or other cured meats. Current evidence suggests it is the nitrite in such foods that causes the headaches.

And it is thought that the lack in some individuals of the enzyme necessary to break down tyramine (which occurs naturally in cheese, chianti wine and yeast) causes headache and other related symptoms. It has further been theorized that inability to break down chemically similar substances found in foods such as chocolates, citrus fruits and bananas may be responsible for migraine in certain individuals. It has been estimated, however, that food is involved in only one of every twenty cases of people who suffer from migraine headache. There are clinics which concern themselves with these painful matters. Perhaps your doctor can direct you to one.

16

AN EATING PLAN FOR ALL

The section on weight and well-being has discussed in detail the relationship between nutrition and your health. That material is now summed up in a comprehensive plan for eating for people of all ages.

In General:

1.   Your weight balance is dependent on the calories you consume and the calories you expend. Like your bank balance, it's a matter of outgo as well as input. And, in and out, calories do count.

2.   A pound of human fat is equivalent to 3,500 calories. Every time, over a period of days, you eat 3,500 calories more than you work and/or exercise off, you gain a pound of fat. If, over another span of days, you do the exact opposite—expend 3,500 calories more than you take in—you lose a pound of fat. The key points to remember: a deficit of 500 calories a day will lose you a pound a week and a deficit of 1,000 calories a day will lose you two pounds a week.

3.   Foods are neither "fattening" nor "nonfattening." They contribute calories to the diet according to their composition and their portion size. A large portion of a "low-calorie" food can contain more calories than a small portion of a "high-

calorie" food. Don't be misled. A weight-reducing diet is not just a list of permitted foods. Most such diets fail because the dieter ignores the size of the portion he's eating. If it says 3 ounces of ground beef, that's what it means. A 6-ounce patty contains twice as many calories.

4. Count every calorie. Your body, be assured, is counting them. Don't ignore "small" snacks, like a cupful of peanuts —800 calories!

5. Remember that you can drink calories as well as eat them. Milk and orange juice are excellent foods, but they do contain calories. So do sugar-free soft drinks and alcoholic beverages which do not contribute any nutrients (two small 2-ounce martinis, for example, are worth 320 calories). Water, on the other hand, is the only thing you consume that has no calories. And water is the most important constituent of the body. It makes up somewhere between 55 and 70 percent of your body weight. The average adult needs five or six glasses of water a day. And the loss of 20 to 22 percent of your total body weight through dehydration can be fatal.

6. Look up a table of caloric contents of foods and drinks.* You will be astonished to find that bread is only 60 calories a slice and that a 3-ounce slice of roast beef, barely enough to cover that slice of bread, has 250 calories! This is not to say that you should not eat roast beef. But you should know the order of magnitude of what you are eating.

7. Don't believe those popular charlatans who try to convince you that you can eat as much protein as you want without ever getting fat. Sources of protein usually are also high in fat. Meat, for example, contains more calories from fat than from protein. Anyway, protein contains 4 calories per gram, just as carbohydrates do. Fat contains 9 calories per gram.

8. Cut down on sugar. A teaspoonful of sugar may be only 20 or 30 calories (depending on how "heaping" it is). But six cups of coffee a day with two teaspoonsful of sugar in each cup amount to 300 calories. That's almost three pounds of body fat a month!

*Jean Mayer, *Overweight: Causes, Cost and Control,* 6th printing (Englewood Cliffs, N. J., Prentice-Hall), 1968 (6th printing 1973)

9.   Look up a table giving you the caloric values of exercise.* Just walking an hour a day is, for example, the equivalent of 250 calories. That's a half a pound a week, thirteen pounds a year.

Adults:

1.   Variety and moderation are the keys to good nutrition. The greater the number of foods in your diet, particularly those not heavily processed, the less the chances you will be deficient in any nutrient. Eat a variety of cereal products, vegetables and fruits, dairy and other animal products.

2.   In an era when hard physical labor is rare, your food intake must be relatively small if you are going to keep your weight where you want it. This is all the more reason why every food you consume should "carry its weight," nutritionally speaking. Avoid eating "empty calories," dishes high in sugar and fat and little or nothing else.

3.   Cardiovascular diseases (those of the heart and blood vessels), strokes and kidney-vascular diseases add up to the Number One health problem in America today. They constitute the leading cause of death in adults (over half of the deaths in men, and a growing proportion in women). And hypertension (high blood pressure) and atherosclerosis (hardening of the arteries) are among the chief causes of disability.

4.   All the evidence we have shows that the higher your blood cholesterol, the higher your chances of developing atherosclerosis. This, in turn, greatly increases your chances of coronary occlusion and stroke. We know also that your blood cholesterol is dependent on four factors: (1) your heredity (over which you have no control); (2) your weight (which should be controlled); (3) your daily activity (which you should probably increase); and (4) the nature of your diet.

Cholesterol in your diet increases your blood cholesterol. For example, two eggs a day, which contain 500 mg. of cholesterol, may increase your blood cholesterol by as much as 25 milligrams per 100 milliliters or even more. Another factor is the amount of fat in your diet. You should try to keep fat down to 30 percent of your calories. Saturated fats—that is, meat fat, hydrogenated vegetable fats, butter fat—increase your choles-terol. On the other hand, polyunsaturated fats—such as those in corn oil, safflower oil, or fish liver oil—reduce it. Mono-unsaturated fats (the main constituents of olive oil) don't affect it too much one way or the other except, as is the case with all fat, they do contribute about 9 calories per gram and should be watched for weight control.

5.   Weight control and regular exercise habits are useful preventers of hypertension. There is also considerable evidence that populations on low-salt diets have far less hypertension than people who eat a lot of salt. So don't wait until your blood pressure reaches a certain figure, say 140/90, before you are placed on a lower-salt intake. Begin using lemon and a great variety of spices as a substitute for heavy salting. It's not only better preventive medicine, it's better cooking!

6.   Eat plenty of fish as a good source of animal protein. It is also low in fat, low in saturated and high in polyun-saturated fat and high in minerals. Try to balance equally at least the number of meals with meat—such as beef or pork—with meals centered on poultry and fish which are much lower in fat.

7.   Fresh fruit and vegetables in season are preferable. But when they are not available, be sure to eat plenty of canned or frozen fruits and vegetables.

8.   Whole-grain cereals and breads are preferable to the enriched varieties. Avoid the highly milled and unenriched bakery products. Remember that bread is a useful, low-fat food, which is not automatically fattening unless you eat too many slices or load it up with fat.

9.   Skim milk and cheese are excellent alternative sources of calcium to whole milk. Remember, the calorie and fat con-tents of cheeses vary widely depending on the type.

10.   Eat a complete diet every day. If you think you want additional insurance against any possible deficiencies, take a multivitamin tablet which provides the Recommended Daily Allowance for all the vitamins required. Do not take massive doses of vitamins which can be dangerous, or "organic" supple-ments which cost a lot of money and have no more value than **169**   the regular kind.

Birth: Pregnancy and Nursing

1.   No period is more important from the viewpoint of nutrition, both for the mother and for the child, than when the mother is literally "eating for two." And yet this is still the most neglected phase of nutrition. A pregnant woman should not gain too much weight, say much over thirty pounds, during the nine months of her confinement. But she should put on two to three pounds a month and in no case less than eighteen pounds. Twenty-four pounds is a good average.

2.   Although a pregnant woman should try to keep up her physical activity, she is, in fact, less active than she normally is, particularly during the last three months. As a result, she will gain the required amount on little more than she ate when she was not pregnant (and more active). This means that if her diet was unsatisfactory before her pregnancy, it can be improved mainly by substituting better foods rather than by adding new ones. Replace "empty calories" by whole-grain cereals, eggs, lean meat and fish, low-fat milk and cheese and plenty of fruits and vegetables.

3.   Unlike the pregnant woman, the nursing mother does need considerably more food than she did before her pregnancy. Whatever she was doing before having the baby, she probably does it now and takes care of the infant besides. In addition, her breasts produce milk, as much as a quart (or more) a day, after nursing is well established. Consequently, a new mother needs extra animal protein (eggs, meat, fish), extra calcium (milk and cheese), extra vitamins and minerals (whole-grain cereal, fruits and vegetables).

4.   Part of the weight gained during pregnancy is reserved for breast-feeding. So remember this: you will lose weight more easily and get back to that girlish figure faster if you breast-feed your baby.

Your Baby:

1.   Breast milk has, of course, been the food of newborn human babies since the beginning of mankind. And there is nothing, despite all our scientific studies and advances, which suggests it is no longer their ideal food. For example, mother's milk is much lower in sodium than cow's milk (and salt may

be of significance in the development of hypertension much later in life). Excessive fatness in the baby (which again may lead to the problem of obesity years later) is less likely to occur in a breast-fed baby.

2. Don't start your baby on solid foods before your pediatrician advises you to. A recent study indicates that most mothers jump the gun in this regard—usually just to keep up with Mrs. Jones. If your pediatrician tells you to start the baby on iron-enriched cereal, for example, this is not a license to start her or him on everything else at once.

3. When your baby is old enough to be on a mixed, solid-food diet, don't continue to believe that the more milk consumed the better. No infant or child needs more than a quart of milk a day. Much more than that—which might be displacing other foods much richer in iron and copper—could lead to anemia.

4. In lieu of "baby foods," you can feed your child foods mashed in an electric blender. However, remember that the prime advantage of baby foods is that they are biologically safe. So if you decide to do-it-yourself, make sure the food is freshly prepared. Also, don't oversalt the food. In fact, since a small baby's taste buds are not yet developed, you don't need to salt it at all.

5. Don't forget the baby's vitamins. If the youngster does not get plenty of fruit juice, he or she needs vitamin C. And also, of course, vitamin D. But only use officially recommended dosages.

The Toddler:

1. Don't be alarmed if, at the age of eighteen months to two years, your small child appears to eat less. She or he is gaining much more slowly than she or he did during the first year. Also, your child is eating adult foods in adult dishes instead of baby food in miniature dishes and, therefore, only seems to eat less than before.

2. Nutrition, whether for the toddler or an older person, is a matter of how much of what foods you eat during the whole day. If a small child seems obviously happier on five meals a day than on three, there is no harm in the two additional snacks.

Just make sure that they are equally nutritious. They need not entail elaborate preparation. Having a toddler in the house does not mean the mother must become a short-order cook on a fifteen-hour shift.

3.   Don't use sweet desserts or snacks as a reward. That's the last thing you want to do for your child's teeth, nutrition and health in general. It will only condition him or her to think of sweet, empty-calorie foods as nutritionally or socially superior. Also, take great care to counter those TV ads which extoll sweetness in candy, cereals, cookies and cakes. Start early and be firm. In fact, go one step further: keep candy and cookies high in sugar out of the house altogether. Use fruits as dessert whenever possible. Don't feed your child sugar-coated cereals, some of which contain more sugar than cereal. Go easy on the sugar on other cereals or on fruit. Avoid high-fat foods as well.

4.   Your toddler is entitled to have some likes and dislikes when it comes to foods. After all, you accept idiosyncrasies in your husband and guests. If he or she does not like meat, just replace the "problem" with fish and eggs, or disliked vegetables by other vegetables and a *variety* of fruit.

5.   Don't use the television as a day-in, day-out babysitter or else your toddler will start off as a sitter and probably remain inactive and a spectator for the rest of his or her life. Get the child to play actively as many hours as possible. Otherwise, you will be creating a potential lifelong health problem.

The Child:

1.   There is no special nutritional virtue in eating at particular times during the day. Children, however, should not be expected to play or study all morning without food. If they will eat a good breakfast, give it to them. Otherwise, prepare a nutritious midmorning snack to eat at home or at school.

2.   Children's physical activity varies widely from day to day, so expect that on some days your youngster will eat more than on others.

3.   Don't force a child to finish everything on his or her plate. This may push him or her toward overweight. Teach children to take helpings small enough that they are sure to eat them. Seconds, if wanted, will be requested.

172

4.   Give your children some say in the planning of menus, but don't cater excessively to their whims. Allow them to replace foods they dislike with other foods in the same category. But don't let them force a lot of additional work on you. Try to develop their taste for a great variety of foods.

5.   Don't let them pass up the nutritious main course and then gorge themselves on dessert. One way to prevent that is just not to serve high-calorie, low-nutrient desserts. Instead, use fruit as much as possible.

6.   There is nothing wrong with snacks for children; just be sure that they're nutritious. A good sandwich is vastly preferable to a piece of cake; a glass of skim milk or fruit juice is always preferable to a soft drink. High-fat or high-sugar snack foods give very poor value, both from the viewpoint of your pocketbook and of child nutrition.

7.   Children need ample vitamin D or they get rickets. They can obtain enough of it if they drink vitamin D–enriched milk or get plenty of sunshine or take a vitamin supplement.

8.   The prevalence of overweight among children is increasing. It is linked much more closely to underexercising than to overeating. When overweight children are compared to those of normal weight, the extra calories going to fat come much more frequently from physical inactivity than from consuming too much food. Get your children to exercise *every day*. If possible, get them to walk to school. If not, perhaps they can walk part of the way. Get them to cultivate those sports such as hiking, tennis and swimming which they can take part in all their lives. Don't drive them to places they could reach by walking or bicycling. And make sure they get plenty of activity during the weekend.

Adolescents:
1.   It is important that adolescents be well fed. Adolescence is a period of rapid growth and heightened activity during which needs for nutrients are uncommonly high. Poor nutrition during this period means that the final growth spurt may be incomplete. It may also mean greater susceptibility to disease, especially tuberculosis.

2.   Forming good food habits during adolescence is of

special significance. Food habits voluntarily acquired during that period are more likely to last through adulthood than those imposed on a child by its parents.

3.   Being fit and *feeling* healthy, fit and attractive during adolescence have advantages that persist throughout life. Recent studies have demonstrated that the "self-image" acquired in youth is likely to be a permanent one, even though one's shape may be altered drastically as one ages. Young people who are (or think they are) too fat during adolescence often feel fat and unattractive when adults, even if by then they have controlled their weight adequately. Fit adolescents are more likely to see later episodes of overweight as no more than temporary handicaps which they can correct themselves.

4.   Because much of the eating done by adolescents takes place between meals it is important to make available to them the ingredients of nutritious snacks: good bread and high-protein spreads or fillers for sandwiches, fruit juices, milk or skim milk. Try to keep handy a bowl of fruit—apples, oranges, other fruit in season. Don't forbid high-sugar or high-fat snacks or soft drinks. Just don't have them in the house. You can generally count on the fact that your adolescents are unlikely to walk to the store to get them.

5.   Most adolescent boys, though perhaps not interested in nutrition and health as such, are intensely interested in fitness, in athletic performance and becoming tall and looking impressive to members of what used to be called the weaker sex. These legitimate longings can be the basis for the acceptance of a wholesome dietary regimen.

6.   Athletic performance is dependent on a sound diet (as well as sufficient rest, the avoidance of cigarettes, and the consumption of plenty of water and other nonalcoholic, preferably nutritious fluids). It is not dependent on the consumption of massive amounts of meat and a low-carbohydrate diet generally, as is still believed by too many coaches. A high-protein diet (which, when you analyze it, is usually a high-fat diet) does not improve performance (in fact, there is some evidence that it may hamper it), and sets the stage for a massive rise of cholesterol in later years.

7.   Adolescent girls are rarely interested in nutrition.

That interest comes later, when they marry and raise children. But adolescent girls and young women are terribly preoccupied with their weight and their looks. The desire to look well may be used to promote a sound diet, not too high in calories, but high enough in nutrients so that their skin, their eyes, their fingernails and their hair will have the glow of health, rather than the dullness of anemia and malnutrition generally.

8. Girls should be persuaded that a sufficient amount of exercise is needed not only for weight control but for the firm look of fitness which is so integral a component of beauty. You can become thin solely through dieting, at some cost in comfort. But you may well be thin and flabby. Exercise as well as "watching one's diet" will make you look lithe and firm for a much more attractive appearance.

9. Recent studies have demonstrated scientifically something which friendly observers had found empirically: girls want to be thinner (by at least two dress sizes) than boys would like them to be. If you are a well-built, fit, attractive size 14, don't try to be a size 12 simply because it is the fashion among models. A Twiggy is attractive to some, but more substantial girls, from the Venus de Milo to Sophia Loren, have had more admirers in the past twenty-five centuries.

10. Parents should remember that adolescent girls are so sensitized to weight problems by television, radio and magazine ads and by the current craze for "dieting" that they can easily go overboard and literally starve themselves to death. Anorexia nervosa is a self-starvation syndrome seen in adolescent girls and young women who see themselves as fat (and refuse to recognize that they are hungry) even when they are in the last stages of emaciation. All too often, this dangerous condition is precipitated by the thoughtless remark of a male important to them: father, favorite uncle, brother or boy friend. Adolescence is in many ways a fragile period. Don't coddle adolescents, but remember that they bruise easily.

Old Age:

1. Older people do not really want to be treated differently from younger people. But the aged have a number of built-in handicaps to good nutrition. First, they have less

money. They may live alone and have no motivation to cook. They may have trouble chewing because they have lost too many teeth or their dentures do not fit. They may have no transportation, or have trouble shopping because of arthritis, partial deafness or poor eyesight. They need your help, even though they will not ask for it. Be tactful and discerning. Do their shopping with them or for them; invite them to eat with you when possible. Investigate community meal plans in their behalf.

2. Old age does not by itself bring about special nutrition problems. But, because elderly people are less active, they need to eat a smaller total amount of food. That means that every calorie must carry its weight in nutrients or deficiencies will occur. Cutting down on sugar, fat and unenriched bakery goods is a wise idea. Keeping up the consumption of milk (or skim milk), cheese, fish, poultry, whole cereals, vegetables and fruits is essential.

3. Because many of the conditions which come with old age are not presently curable, the elderly are targets for charlatans who can promise "cures" where no physician could. Help protect the older people from the claims of miracle merchants who sell extraordinary "health" foods through extravagant claims. Money spent on such overpraised items would be better used on less expensive food at the supermarket, on dental care, on legitimate medical attention, or on recreation.

4. Above all, remember that, as the child is the father of the man, the middle-aged man is the father of the elderly. What happens to your nutrition and health in old age is very much the result of the practices and preparations of your preceding years.

3

THE
MARKET
AND
THE
KITCHEN

17 FADS, FAKES AND FALLACIES

There used to be a popular joke about how everything that's fun in life is either illegal, immoral or fattening. In today's more complicated times, the literal-minded would feel compelled to add "or bad for your heart, liver, lungs, genes, brain and bones."

The problem is more than just the menace of the nasty habits, such as smoking or drinking, you innocently acquired before you knew the facts; it is that you can't even do the things necessary to life without endangering life. At least you can't if you believe all the toxicologists, ecologists, consumer-protection groups, food crusaders, research scientists and various other professional and amateur improvers of the quality of living.

You can't breathe deeply in certain places at certain times; you mustn't exercise too strenuously or too little; and reproducing your own kind is fraught with genetic peril.

Most terrifying of all is sitting down to a good meal.

An intelligent person who reads the papers, keeps up with current science, and takes life at all seriously must eye each plateful or glassful critically, but still may be thoroughly at sea in distinguishing "true" from "false" from "exaggerated" in the following statements:

Cow's milk: Its fat will cause heart disease; its lactose makes you blind. Contains DDT. [Exaggerated; false; false.]

Mother's milk: Contains so much DDT that, if bottled, it would not be permitted to cross state lines. [False.]

Eggs: High in cholesterol; could give you a coronary. [Partly true for certain individuals.]

White bread, spaghetti, macaroni, etc: Made of flour deficient in nutrients. Most vitamins and minerals removed by milling, and only a few restored through the "enrichment" process. [Partly true.]

Whole-wheat bread: Has a few more nutrients, may retain more pesticides. [Partly true; false.]

Brown rice: Same as whole-wheat bread. And also high in mercury. [Exaggerated; false.]

Meat: High-fat content will give you heart disease. Contaminated by estrogens, which are carcinogenic and interfere with sex function. Lower in nutritive value, since animals are fed devitalized, chemically grown feeds. [Exaggerated; true, but danger unproven; false.]

Sausages and lunch meats: Same as above. High in nitrates, nitrites and other dangerous chemicals. [Exaggerated; true, but danger unproven.]

Fish: Contaminated with mercury, DDT and other toxicants. [Exaggerated.]

Shellfish: Veritable "Typhoid Marys" and sources of infectious hepatitis. Contaminated with oil and pesticides. [Exaggerated.]

Breakfast cereals: Contain either "empty calories" or fill you up with "synthetic chemicals." Added sugar may promote diabetes. [Partly true.]

Butter, hydrogenated vegetable fats: Raise your blood cholesterol, give you heart disease. [True.]

Polyunsaturated oils: Rumored to cause multiple sclerosis and cancer. [False.]

Vegetables and fruits: Contaminated by pesticides, some of which are related to nerve gas. [Exaggerated to false.]

Water: Full of chemicals, including fluorine, which will harden your skull and soften your brain. [Exaggerated to ridiculous.]

Coffee: Promotes diabetes and coronaries. Keeps you awake nights. [Probably mostly exaggerated; true for some people.]

Ice cream: High in fat (heart disease) and in sugar (empty calories, diabetes), possibly flavored with cancer-causing chemicals. [Partly true.]

Salt: Promotes high blood pressure. [True.]

Liver: A veritable repository of DDT, parathion and artificial estrogens. [Exaggerated.]

Cheeses: Full of heart-threatening fat and cholesterol. [Exaggerated.]

Yogurt: Makes rats blind (if they eat nothing else). [True.]

Canned foods: Devitalized, low in nutrients, filled with chemical preservatives and antioxidants. [False.]

Frozen foods: Changes in store and home-freezer temperatures will bring about "bacterial infestation." [True, but unlikely.]

Obviously a good deal of the above is nonsense, either because the proposition was untrue to start with or because its truth is carried to a ridiculous extreme.

And you, if taking the above literally, have every right to demand:

Isn't there anything left to eat?

There is more to eat than ever. The greater your choice of foods, the less chance you will miss out on essential nutrients. Eat as many unprocessed foods as you can. Eat fresh foods in season. Wash them well before serving.

Canned and frozen vegetables and fruits are useful foods. They enable you to provide a varied diet when fresh foods are out of season.

"Convenience foods" are fine. But your family will eat better if you prepare the food yourself. The simpler the preparation, the better the nutrition.

Choose leaner cuts of *meat.* When eating, trim fat. Liver and organ meats are particularly lean. Bacon is relatively expensive and fat. If you must have bacon, Canadian is leaner and nutritionally superior.

White bread is a low-fat food. Although enriched bread and bakery products are lower in some trace minerals and vitamins than whole grain, they contain essential nutrients which you may not get elsewhere.

Milk and *cheese* are still the major sources of calcium.

Eggs are a near-ideal food for many people, particularly children, adolescent girls and pregnant or lactating women.

It seems reasonable in cooking to replace saturated fats with polyunsaturated oils. Don't overcook them, however.

I can find nothing good, nutritionally, to say about *sugar*. The calories are present, but the nutrients are not. And the difference between a good and bad diet is how much of the nutrients you get with the calories.

Carefully read *labels* on jars, cans, boxes and other packages. They're becoming (at last!) more informative as to ingredients and calorie content.

Our rich and varied agriculture and advanced food technology make it possible to provide a highly nutritious diet for your family, provided we make the proper choices. Modern sanitation has practically eliminated any *danger* of disease-carrying organisms in industrially prepared canned food, and considerably decreased it in most other foods. Pollutants are carefully monitored not only by federal and state agencies but also by many scientific and industrial organizations, and it appears that in the past few years episodes of contamination have been picked up early, before the food reached the consumer.

Is there any way for us to help continue this reassuring work?

Continue to press for expanded investigation of environmental risks, for the development of more nutritious processed foods and drinks, and for more informative labeling. (See Chapter 19.) All of us should try also to distinguish between real problems, unsupported claims, and the mouthings of food cranks. Otherwise there may soon be a national tendency to eat nothing but bean sprouts and alfalfa, on which a few deluded souls have already undertaken to survive.

My son came home from school, and as he sat at the dinner table, he cast a disdainful eye on the roast and announced he had become a vegetarian. What could have brought this about?

His motivation may be compassion (why should we kill other animals to feed ourselves?) or it may be imaginary health reasons (meat causes cancer). Or it could be an Oriental philosophy (the Zen Buddhist way of eating is necessary for longevity and rejuvenation).

We told the boy to stop being ridiculous and to eat his meat. He responded by declaring that only insensitive persons endowed with the grossest type of sensuality would eat meat. All he wanted was some rice or nuts or beans. Isn't there anything we can do to change his attitude?

The direct order, which you unsuccessfully tried, is likely to be, in contemporary jargon, counterproductive. It might be more useful if you or your husband were to conduct a calm, interested conversation after the meal to determine how far the young man plans to deviate from the normal eating pattern, and why.

The danger to the youngster—and thus the extent of the need for parental intervention—varies enormously. It depends on whether he has become a convinced but sensible vegetarian who mildly limits his diet or whether he has fallen for the truly hazardous extremes of the Zen macrobiotic diet.

Are there several different types of vegetarians among boys and girls?

Many young people just do not like red meat. They will, however, eat poultry, fish or eggs. Although their diet becomes more vegetarian than otherwise, it is far from completely so. The situation raises absolutely no nutritional problem because the known nutrients in beef, lamb, and pork they're refusing are present also in the foods they're accepting.

Quite often the young person is horrified at innocent animals being driven to the slaughterhouse to satisfy the appetites of the human species which could easily feed itself in other ways. Most vegetarians animated by such convictions are in no way averse to drinking milk or to eating nonfertile eggs. They are classified as "ovo-lacto-vegetarians."

Are there nutrients lacking in the diets of these people?

As far as we know, this type of diet provides perfectly satisfactory nutrition. With plenty of milk and cheese and eggs every day, meat will in no way be missed. Protein, calcium, B_2, iron and trace minerals will be present in quite sufficient amounts in the diet. Exhaustive studies of Seventh-Day Adventists, who are ovo-lacto-vegetarians, have repeatedly shown them to be in excellent health.

But what if our son has embraced complete vegetarianism?

If he refuses any animal food whatsoever, there may be problems. As long as he is ready to have a varied vegetarian diet —with beans, nuts, whole-grain cereals and plenty of fruits and vegetables—the most serious risk is not, as you might think, lack of protein. The real problem is vitamin B_{12} deficiency. In the long run, if allowed to go uncorrected, it portends a severe danger.

An extensive study of a group of British vegetarians revealed that a number of them exhibited a form of incurable disease, combined subacute degeneration of the spinal nerves, due to a deficiency of vitamin B_{12}. Calcium, vitamin D and some trace minerals, such as chromium, may also be low in an all-vegetable diet.

If your child persists in following such a diet, try to get him to compromise by eating nonfertile eggs or at least (like Gandhi) milk and cheese. If you cannot negotiate this arrangement, he must have a daily vitamin pill containing vitamin B_{12}.

Extreme, vehement vegetarianism, omitting milk, may also suggest a deep-seated psychological difficulty. If even milk is outlawed by the regimen your son is following, it would be a good idea to seek the advice of your family doctor or the school psychiatrist.

Are there other unusual opinions about food encountered today among young people?

A fear of additives and of various unnamed poisons is pushing some boys and girls to eat fewer and fewer staple foods.

In some cases, the fear is based on a specific, often erroneous, belief. Boys, for instance, may be afraid that female sex hormones, which they believe are still used in treating meat, will sap their maleness. DES has been essentially withdrawn, and was never present in amounts large enough to influence their sex characteristics. If no deep personality disturbance is present, they can be reassured without too much difficulty.

What current dietary fad do you regard as most dangerous?

The most harmful package of notions I know of is expressed by rigid adherence to the macrobiotic diet. This so-called long-life regimen was concocted by a now-deceased Japanese named Sakurazawa Nyoiti, known in the Western world as George Ohsawa. His curious mixture of Asiatic philosophy and biochemical terminology seems to hold great attraction for young people who have little knowledge of Eastern metaphysics and even less of biochemistry.

This doctrine is based on the principle of yin-yang—antagonistic but complementary forces.

Yin, we are told, is centrifugal, producing silence, calmness, cold and darkness. In nutrition it is associated with vegetables, salads, vitamin C, and sweet, sour and hot foods.

Yang is centripetal and heavy, producing sound, action, heat and light. In nutrition it is associated with animal food, cereal, salt and vitamins A, D and K.

Yin foods are tropical or grow in the summer. Yang foods grow in the winter and are frigid.

Do you, as a professional nutritionist, believe any of the contentions of Ohsawa?

Not a bit! And their general absurdity would not be alarming to me except for one thing: the highest goal is slowly to divest one's diet of everything but unpolished rice.

The macrobiotic dieter achieves this ultimate by moving progressively through ten different diets numbered from minus three to plus seven, each one more and more limited. The first two or three diets are heavy on rice, but they still contain some animal protein and are nutritionally balanced. For example, the first includes 30 percent vegetables, 30 percent animal foods, and 15 percent salads and fruits.

185

By the fourth diet, salads and fruits have dropped out and animal foods are down to 10 percent. The sixth diet no longer includes any animal foods. The further you go, the more deficient the diets become. As the disciple "progresses," he eliminates all animal foods and more and more vegetables. And his diet becomes more and more dangerous, with no vitamin B_{12} and soon no vitamin A, C or D. The ultimate goal is the tenth diet, consisting of 100 percent unpolished rice.

What's the matter with rice?

Rice is a perfectly good food when it is included in a varied diet. But a diet of rice alone obviously lacks a number of vital nutrients. For young people with little or no understanding of nutrition, the lure of yin-yang is bolstered by pages and pages of food classifications, technical sounding discussions of water content and the like, and great varieties of recipes that are supposed to be medically useful.

Even if the medical proposals are more or less without value, there isn't anything harmful about them, is there?

Wait till you hear them! Paranoia is treated by diet No. 7 and rheumatism by grilled rice only. No. 7 is also recommended for meningitis, neurasthenia, obesity, ear infections, peritonitis, poliomyelitis ("a very yin sickness") and schizophrenia. Syphilis, Ohsawa maintained, is "contagious only for those who have a yin constitution," and is easy to cure "since the spirochete that causes syphilis is very yin, therefore weak and vulnerable to salt." The familiar refrain "Try diet No. 7" is not very reassuring to those of us who are alarmed by the explosive increase in syphilis cases, especially among the young.

It certainly seems that the macrobiotic diet is extremely dangerous nonsense. What kind of person do you think George Ohsawa was?

He probably was a nice man. He wrote enthusiastically about tolerance, good humor, goodwill toward men and the need to divest ourselves of greed. But all this should not blind us to the fact that his call, if followed faithfully, is that of a Pied Piper who can lead young people to a totally inappropriate and miserable death.

If it turns out that my son has become not one of the moderate enthusiasts for vegetarianism but a "gung-ho" addict of the macrobiotic diet, what can I do about it?

Your youngster must, just as rapidly as possible, be brought back to nutritional variety. Perhaps he needs counseling in other ways as well.

Parents may not be the best people to conduct this re-education. A younger, very wise person, who is liked and trusted by your son, would be an ideal choice for the assignment.

Professional help, a physician, perhaps a psychiatrist who is learned about nutrition, might be needed. You shouldn't make a mountain out of a molehill. But a larger risk is to see a real mountain and dismiss it as a molehill.

Such athletes as boxers are frequently put on crash diets to make them eligible for lower weight classifications. Is this a safe procedure?

Crash diets to cut weight are always dangerous. When weight is lost, all sorts of sensitive mechanisms have to make precise adjustments to the changed demands on them. A sudden contrived drop in weight can disturb these mechanisms and bring on serious illnesses. And, when they can do that, at very least they can put the boxer at a disadvantage when he climbs through the ropes and into the ring.

A few years ago there was a lot of publicity about physicians who successfully reduced the weights of hospitalized obese patients by the total deprivation of food. This seems to be one way to go about it. Is it a good way?

Obviously, someone who isn't getting anything to eat is going to lose weight, a lot of weight. I cannot conceive an effort of this sort being carried out except under extreme circumstances. If the very life of a patient were being put in immediate jeopardy by reason of his obesity, total fasting might be indicated. This might be a patient whose fatness might make impossible seriously needed surgery.

Some coaches and trainers believe it is wise to prepare an
athlete for a strenuous event by putting him on a diet more

than ordinarily high in fat content. Is there any wisdom in this?

There is not. The notion behind it is based on the fact that fat yields about twice as many calories per gram as does carbohydrate. This suggests erroneously that fat provides about twice the available energy that carbohydrate does. Actually the significant factor is that carbohydrate yields more calories per liter of oxygen than does the burning of fat.

I have no uncontrollable enthusiasm for special diets for athletes.

I've just read an advertisement for liquid vitamin E. It said it would help clear up skin problems, reduce wrinkles, and that it was excellent for stretch marks. A half-ounce costs $7.95. Is liquid vitamin E, applied directly, effective in treating skin problems?

Save your money. This is just one in a long list of benefits erroneously ascribed to vitamin E. Many of the claims are interpretations from animal studies, the results of which have never been successfully duplicated in man. In some cases, as in this one, the basis is even more questionable. Actually, a deodorant containing vitamin E has been withdrawn from production at FDA urging, after it had received a great many complaints of severe underarm rashes.

Vitamin E does play a role in various body functions related particularly to fat intake, but that role is still very much under investigation. The Recommended Daily Allowance is 15 International Units. A normal diet containing whole grains, leafy vegetables, and vegetable oils will give you an ample supply.

Are nuts really a good source of nutrients. Are nuts sold in health food stores better than the kind you buy in supermarkets?

To your first question, a qualified yes. Nuts are moderately good foods, but they're high in calories. One cup of Brazil nuts yields 900 calories, a cup of roasted peanuts 800. They vary widely in protein, fat and mineral content. None contain more than traces of vitamins A and C. All are low in calcium. Some, such as almonds, are good sources of vitamin B_2, others are low.

Some, such as walnuts, are good sources of polyunsaturated fats; others not.

Eating salted nuts unnecessarily increases your sodium intake, which you don't need, particularly if you're middle-aged.

All in all, nuts are a pleasant component of your diet, but they're no panacea. They don't allow you to pass by milk or cheese, vegetables and other fruits.

Nuts sold in health stores are identical to those sold in supermarkets. Even if you are panicked about pesticides, they can hardly penetrate the shell of a walnut. The type of fertilizer doesn't enter into the question, either. One would hardly put horse manure around a walnut tree.

An advertisement in a drugstore trade journal announced: "Now you can make money from all those health nuts" and described an introductory deal with a profit of 40 percent. This kind of markup is the rule in specialty stores, not in supermarkets. The latter make money on large volumes and small markups. The lesson to the buyer should be self-evident.

Just what is meant by the term "organic foods"? I seem to see the organic label on an increasing number of foods.

Unfortunately, I can't define them for you, and neither can anyone else exactly. Asked for a definition, a large supplier of so-called organic foods said that, like all "organic compounds" they contain carbon. But so do all other foods.

Consumers mistakenly believe that all "organic foods" are produced without pesticides and artificial fertilizers and that they are free of preservatives, hormones and antibiotics. But there are no legal standards or regulations. Therefore, growers or processors or retailers may apply the "organic" rubber stamp wherever they please with complete freedom. And, of course, they charge more for "organic foods."

In one study, foods bearing the "organic" label cost between one-and-a-half to twice as much as their counterparts in the supermarket. In general, the difference in price was found to be greater for processed items such as cereal, pasta and bread than for unprocessed items such as produce, poultry and eggs.

Recently, legislation has been introduced in various states

legally to define "organically grown" and "organically processed" foods. This legislation would also set up a governmental system of monitoring organic farming and processing. Until such legislation becomes a reality, however, "organic" foods are what the seller says they are.

Am I correct in assuming that natural or "organic" vitamins are no better than regular vitamins?

You are correct. The idea of selling natural vitamins as somehow better is a hoax. A vitamin is nothing more than a specific compound, whether it is synthesized or extracted from a plant. The only difference is that those from "natural" sources seem to cost more.

I was interested in a product on the nature food store shelf called choline. Is choline effective in keeping fat from accumulating in the liver and arteries?

Choline manufacturers and nature food store proprietors might have a difficult time explaining why any normal person should swallow choline pills. Choline, widely available in the diet and manufactured in the body, is generally considered to be an essential nutrient, although a deficiency has never been demonstrated in man.

It has been observed in experimental animals. One of the symptoms is fatty liver. Although choline has been widely used to treat fatty liver, as well as cirrhosis and hepatitis, its therapeutic effect has never been demonstrated.

The claim that choline controls atherosclerosis is probably linked to the fact that it is a constituent of lecithin. And lecithin has unfortunately and erroneously been popularized by food faddists as effective in lowering blood cholesterol.

While there is considerable interest in choline among researchers at present, there is as yet no basis for recommending it as a preventive measure.

You seem to be putting down the health food stores. I have never met more concerned people than those who work in these stores. They go out of their way to help you select the supplement which most closely meets your needs. Have you ever been in a health food store? You ought to try it.

I have visited a number of health food stores. I must agree with you that the employees tend to be accessible, gracious and anxious to help. And they're right there with advice. But their counsel is not better (in fact, probably far less sensible) than that of your mother-in-law. The employee, without any medical or nutritional credentials, is willing to do what no good practicing physician would be presumptuous enough to do: make a diagnosis and prescribe treatment without a medical evaluation.

So it is that each year millions of dollars' worth of dolomite, sea salt, kelp, bone meal, as well as a variety of vitamin and mineral supplements which may range in effect from useless to hazardous, are sold to individuals genuinely interested in good health.

It would be far sounder for you to find yourself a physician to evaluate your health or a dietician to improve your nutrition. They will prescribe only what is necessary. Don't confuse courtesy with knowledge or wisdom.

Is it useful for a dieter to include in his eating program such things as wheat germ and brewer's yeast?

Wheat germ and brewer's yeast are useful foods, but have no particular magic virtue. A good diet with a sufficient variety of food is going to be balanced without such exotic supplements. Live yeast, incidentally, may use up more vitamins in the intestine than it actually provides, and thus its consumption may be self-defeating.

Is the extrapolation of animal experiments to people without any sound basis for doing so a common error?

It is a typical one into which nutrition faddists fall. Some misguided young mothers today, for example, are starving as they try to subsist on fresh grass and powdered alfalfa while they nurse their undernourished babies on "the same diet that helps cows produce a lot of milk."

The theory seems to make sense, but it overlooks the fact that the cow ruminates, while the human mother does not. The cow incubates in one of her four stomachs some fifty to seventy-five pounds of bacteria that digest grass and make it nutritionally available to herself and her babies. For a woman to try

191

living on alfalfa makes no more sense than for people to take huge amounts of vitamin E because a deficiency of it lowers the reproductive rate of guinea pigs.

Are there rules we can use to enable us to spot fads and faddists?

1. Beware of any "magic" food supplement that purports to solve all your health problems.

2. Only a faddist will promise to prevent or cure diseases that physicians generally regard as incurable.

3. If someone promises easy solutions (which may defy the laws of nature) to difficult problems, he or she is likely to be a faddist.

4. Faddists often recognize only one problem or only one factor in a complex problem at a time. (A study at Boston's Peter Bent Brigham Hospital showed that very low carbohydrate "reducing" diets do elevate blood cholesterol, even when one drinks plenty of water, but the faddists would have you believe otherwise.)

5. Faddists frequently place great emphasis on blood sugar as an indicator of health and mental sanity or the absence thereof.

6. Other faddists operate on the notion that if 1 is good, 100 must be 100 times better. (It can be harmful—fatally so!)

7. Faddists insist that all or most supermarket foods are devitalized, because they are deficient in, among other things, "trace minerals."

8. Faddists would like you to believe that additives are all bad, indeed, deadly.

9. Faddists would have you believe that anything "natural" is splendid for you and anything that isn't is bad.

18 BACTERIA AND SUCH

Our country is on a great back-to-nature kick. Technology of any kind is out, and we are urged to go back to coarse bread, raw milk and raisins from grapes untreated by any of the fungicides. There are fears—unfounded—that there's a massive plot to poison us with constant dosages of food additives. Certainly, there is a refusal to believe that any food additive may actually increase the (bacteriological) safety of a food. Above all, we are exhorted to repudiate what early man believed to be the mythical gods' greatest gift to man: fire.

Cooking food (or pasteurizing milk), some people now say, destroys "the vital principles, the natural vitamins," and, obviously, the mystical aura of simplicity. If, in the words of a ringing TV commercial, "It is not nice to fool Mother Nature," it is clearly even worse to tamper with her by cooking.

People tend to assume that all foods are more nutritious raw than cooked. They aren't. Many believe, often to their regret, that "natural" is a synonym for "pure." In fact, one of the important reasons for cooking food is not for taste or tenderness, but for protection against bacteria and parasites which may contaminate even the most lovingly grown "organic foods."

Of course, there is much good to be said for raw or natural foods. The health-and-wholesomeness movement and our eager efforts at girth control have led people to eat not only more raw carrots and tomatoes but also raw onions, cucumber slices, celery, spinach, cauliflower, mushrooms, turnips, horseradishes and zucchini. A greater variety of fruits are appearing at dessert time as substitutes for calorically heavy cakes and pies.

This is excellent. Raw fruits and vegetables are, in general, better sources of vitamins and minerals than cooked ones. I say "in general" because unlike the gastrointestinal tracts of cattle, goats, horses and rabbits, our gastrointestinal tracts do not harbor the microorganisms that can break the cellulose walls of raw vegetables, converting them to utilizable food and giving us access to the nutrients within. Soft, squishy fruits and vegetables are easily digested and are better sources of nutrients, but harder, cellulose-rich vegetables like cauliflower, spinach and, yes, carrots, are often better digested when they have been cooked.

Cooking with little water and little exposure to air minimizes the loss of nutrients. Saving the cooking water for soup stock is another way to preserve vitamins and minerals.

Grains and seeds are essentially undigested unless ground and cooked. Baking bread or cooking rice doesn't delete nutrients: that happens mostly in the milling (if too thorough).

As a nutritionist, I care about nutrients in the diet. But as a public health man, I am much more worried about the growing neglect of the most elementary precepts of food sanitation. Americans were shocked to learn of the "filth guidelines" of the Food and Drug Administration. These rules, hastily renamed "guidelines for unavoidable defects in food," specify the number of rodent pellets and hair and the number of insect fragments, larvae or eggs allowable for each class of processed foods. Unprocessed foods are equally contaminated. We are, as in the past, in competition for our nourishment with rodents, insects and various microorganisms.

But are not "organic" foods free of pollution?

They may escape chemical pollution but biologically speaking they tend to be the most contaminated of all. Organic fertilizers of animal or human origin are conspicuously the most likely to contain gastrointestinal parasites. In fact, in many underdeveloped areas (Korea is the latest example) widespread infections have been eliminated decisively by switching from age-old fertilizing methods to chemical fertilizers.

Salmonella, which causes more stomach aches than probably anything else, is a frequent inhabitant of the gastrointestinal tract of animals and men. It represents a serious threat if foods are neither washed nor cooked.

Then do you rule out all raw foods from human consumption?

I offer one major rule: any fruit or vegetable eaten raw and unpeeled ought to be washed thoroughly. (In fact, if it is heavily waxed, as are many apples, green peppers and cucumbers, it should be peeled.)

Washing is a particularly useful practice if you use "organic" foods. At an organic farm in California I encountered the belief that "washing takes the goodness away from vegetables." That's especially alarming because a number of Vietnam veterans work on that particular organically fertilized garden. These returned veterans have brought into the country a good many cases of amebiasis, an intestinal infection which is difficult to eliminate and is easily transmitted through contaminated vegetables.

I am constantly astonished to find that a greater and greater number of young people believe that the only reason for washing fruits and vegetables that are to be consumed raw is to eliminate pesticides. Apparently they have forgotten that the major danger in eating is still preeminently bacterial or parasitic contamination.

Does eating raw, unwashed fruits and vegetables constitute the major danger?

No. Dangers are multiplied with animal food. One of the follies of the new era of faddism is the belief that raw milk is superior to pasteurized milk. Raw milk is said to be a source of mysterious nutrients that are otherwise destroyed by pasteurization. It is believed also somehow to escape any blame in the relationship of milk fat to blood cholesterol.

Do not believe any of this. Even if pasteurization did cause a significant loss in nutrients (which doesn't appear to be the case), that disadvantage would be more than canceled out by the major advantage of pasteurization: the elimination of the risk of tuberculosis and other milk-borne infections.

Tuberculosis was for a long time the major cause of condemnation of cattle. (At one time, up to 85 percent of the cattle in one county were infected.) Because the disease agent had an affinity for the human spine, it was responsible for a large number of hunch-back children and adults. Though the tuberculosis-eradication program has met with considerable success, I see little point in betting your children's spines that the raw milk you drink is safe.

Is tuberculosis the only possible menace in raw milk?

The *Brucella* organism, which is eliminated by pasteurization, is the agent of another serious disease, undulant fever. Again, the disease, which brings with it rheumatic pains and the swelling of joints and the spleen, is far less prevalent now than it once was. This is not a sufficient reason for taking an unnecessary chance.

Nor does switching to raw goat milk, as some "organic" communes are doing, eliminate all risk. Goat milk is a carrier of such diseases as Malta fever or brucellosis as well as an equally good breeding ground for pathogenic bacteria of all types. Goat milk (or goat cheese) ought to be pasteurized if it is going to be safe for human consumption, especially for babies.

Thus, I offer another major rule: *drink pasteurized milk.* Don't let anyone convince you that your fear of raw milk (particularly if it comes from a herd and a farm you know nothing about) is unreasonable and reflects only your "square" upbringing.

Eggs represent another hazard. They have often been a cause of salmonellosis if they came from infected birds. If you have to use them raw in eggnogs, wash the shell carefully and never use a cracked egg.

Whatever your grandfather thought about it, don't make a practice of sucking raw eggs. You lose nothing nutritionally by boiling the egg or poaching it, both good ways to keep fat and caloric content within bounds.

Do you approve of the current enthusiasm for eating raw ground meat?

This is one of the riskiest present-day fads and it appears to be spreading. This practice, an enthusiasm of Attila the Hun, was sent back in 451 A.D. across the Rhine, to the lasting benefit of French cooking.

The custom of eating raw meat in the Western world died except in a few remote bastions of the intelligentsia, who apparently took a perverse delight in identifying with their opposites through the consumption of "steak tartare." The Harvard Faculty Club, for example, acquired whatever culinary notoriety it has, through the serving of raw, ground horse steak.

The consumption of raw hamburger (which incidentally does *not* give you any better nutrition than well-cooked meat) is accompanied by serious health risks. American beef is not inspected for tapeworm (which is designated by the euphonious name *Taenia saginata*).

The risk is often compounded by the fact that butchers frequently use the same knives and grinders for both beef and pork. Often, a little ground pork is added to ground beef to improve the flavor. In fact, in the market closest to my laboratory, a sign at the butcher counter recommends such a mixture. At more enlightened shops, a sign cautions customers about the need for thorough cooking of all pork and pork products.

Anyway, the mere fact that the same tools are used for beef and pork means that you may run the risk not only of *Taenia saginata* but also of the pork tapeworm, *Taenia solium*. More dangerous still, of course, is the risk of trichinosis, a dread condition for which there is no cure.

Are there other risks associated with the consumption of raw meat?

There's also toxoplasmosis, caused by a microscopic crescent-shaped organism so tiny you can fit thousands of them on the head of a pin. Among a few unlucky individuals the disease runs wild, causing blindness or neurological damage simulating strokes.

197

A pregnant woman should be particularly careful to avoid raw or undercooked meat. The baby she is carrying may become infected, resulting in birth defects or, years later, bewildering symptoms.

Beyond the risk of these particular parasites, there's the general risk of bacterial contamination. Slaughterhouses are not the most hygienic places in the world. A great many samples of raw meat have been found to be infected with *Clostridium perfringens,* a bacterium often responsible for disease outbreaks. Even more dangerous, many raw meat samples are contaminated with staphylococci of various types which cause acute intestinal disturbance within one to four hours after eating.

If the contaminated meat has been allowed to remain at room temperature for four hours or longer (and you have no way of knowing how much of a head start the meat had before you prepared that steak tartare), enough toxin may be produced to cause serious gastrointestinal upsets. Toxins produced by *Clostridium perfingens* and *Staphylococcus aureus* are not destroyed when such food is cooked, even though the bacteria themselves are killed.

Can you give me some more information about safeguarding against salmonella infection? I understand it's quite common.

Salmonellosis is indeed one of the major causes of foodborne illness. It affects an estimated 2 million Americans a year. The symptoms, which include headache, fever, stomach cramps, diarrhea and vomiting, fortunately are short-lived. The disease, however, can be more serious, particularly in children and the aged.

In certain cases, infected individuals become "carriers" of salmonella bacteria and can be a source of infection for others. Because of this, food-service employees should have regular checkups to insure that they are salmonella-free.

Salmonella organisms can be present in a wide variety of foods, including fresh meat, poultry, fish and eggs. And there is no way to detect it. A few simple precautions, however, can help protect your family against infection.

First, avoid eating raw meat, poultry, fish and eggs. When

cooking, use at least 140 degrees for 10 minutes. (At higher temperatures, foods can be safely cooked in shorter periods.)

Second, thaw frozen meat, fish and poultry slowly by placing them in the refrigerator, not by leaving them out on the kitchen counter.

Third, always use clean platters and utensils when serving these foods. Reuse of platters and utensils from infected raw foods can recontaminate the cooked food.

Fourth, to avoid contamination of other foods, keep one cutting board aside for meat, fish and poultry and another for cutting all other foods.

It is encouraging to note that methods are currently being sought to inhibit the multiplication of salmonella in the food supply. Until such an additive is found and tested for safety, we must rely on good kitchen techniques to provide a defense.

Why do manufacturers, bakers, and other food processors pour, stir or sprinkle into their products some, often many, unfamiliar chemicals with names that are frequently unpronounceable and, occasionally, intimidating?

Preservatives are added for reasons that almost always are clearly justified. Food often has a long way to travel from its point of origin to your dining room table. And it mustn't be permitted to spoil. Chemical additives are included in many foods to prevent it.

Other additives put needed nutrients in the mix—vitamins and minerals, usually. Still more provide color, flavor and stability. The rationale for these is often far less compelling. If these chemicals did not exist or were not used, the cost of the product would often be higher. People would have to be used to less colorful maraschino cherries or orange peels, something which they could stand but which Americans seem reluctant to do.

In general, one can agree that the benefit-to-risk ratio should be the major factor in determining the use of additives. In the case of preservatives, the ratio is very high. In the case of dyes, it is far less compelling.

What with frequent headlines touching on the alleged dangers of certain additives, I keep running into people who profess to believe that there's a massive plot afoot to poison the population of the United States. Are there good reasons for these fears?

There are not. Our food supply today is much safer than it was in the past. Spoilage and microbe infestation once exposed the public to the constant threat of gastroenteritis, not to mention typhoid, cholera, tuberculosis and a variety of other food-borne diseases.

Still, we can expect a great deal of continued controversy over the safety of many specific additives. This will occur partly because some countries have imposed restrictions on certain chemicals that are permitted in the United States. Why? Different countries have different laws and different procedures and, of course, different officials have different opinions.

Anyway, just what is an additive? In a sense, sugar is. So is salt. So are the other condiments. There are, literally, hundreds of lesser-known compounds being added to our food. Let us review the main varieties of additives—it being understood that the fact of our describing them does not necessarily mean that we unconditionally approve of the use of all of them.

Why do some food processors put such chemicals as sulfur dioxide and hydrogen peroxide in the food we are going to eat?

Because of the vastness of our country and the desire of the population to eat any food regardless of the season, the use of preservatives is widespread. Unlike many other kinds of additives, preservatives such as these have an obvious nutritional usefulness in that they help make possible a greater variety and abundance of foods.

One group of chemicals prolongs the "keeping quality" of food by preventing contamination by bacteria or fungi. Some of these substances, sulfur dioxide, sulfites and hydrogen peroxide have been around for decades. This does not by any means guarantee their safety. There is a vast amount of research going on to evaluate the effects of these compounds on the body.

What useful function do antibiotics perform when they become part of the ingredients of a particular food?

Antibiotics used to be added to fish, meat and poultry to retard spoilage. This is still done in certain countries, such as the Soviet Union. When this is done, the product is usually chilled or frozen, and the eventual cooking procedure should destroy any antibiotic authorized as a food preservative. This precaution is taken because unknown doses of antibiotics can kill off some of the body's intestinal bacteria, thus affecting the health in unknown ways. Because of this danger, many countries, the United States in particular, have now placed restrictions on the use of antibiotics.

The group of preservatives known as antioxidants prevents the spoilage of fat and protects taste by inhibiting the formation of dangerous peroxides. Antioxidants also preserve the content of the fat in polyunsaturated fatty acids and fat-soluble vitamins, an obvious nutritional value.

They may even have a worthy side effect. Recent experiments showed that mice fed generous doses of antioxidants live longer.

Acid is a word that scares a lot of people. Yet citric acid, tartaric acid, carbonic acids and other acids are put in some foods. Why?

Acids give added tartness to certain foods and beverages. Tartaric acid, citric acid and lactic acid are mixed in fruit and fruit-juice preparations. Acetic acid, less forbidding in dilution when it's called vinegar, is used in pickling, salads, and relishes. Carbonic acid makes beverages effervescent.

Bases, which are substances which react with acids, are used in baking and to neutralize the increased acidity of certain canned products.

Other flavor additives often have as many as ten or fifteen ingredients. They are widely used in confectionary, alcoholic and nonalcoholic beverages, syrups, ice cream and various other desserts. Their safety is under constant examination. Now that cyclamates, which caused tumors to develop in experimental rats, have been banned, saccharin is the main alternative to sugar. It has been used since the last century, and its safety in normal dosage was confirmed by the National Academy of Sciences, though a daily limit was put on its use. There has recently been an effort to reinstate cyclamate, and there are periodic reports of harm done by saccharin, but so far neither the status of cyclamate nor that of saccharin has been altered.

What, in particular, was believed to be wrong with monosodium glutamate? And what is its current status?

The taste enhancer, MSG, was in the news as a result of studies which showed that injections and stomach-fed doses of the chemical caused structural changes in the brains of infant mice, rats, rabbits and a rhesus monkey. This dangerous side effect seems to be limited to infant mammals and not to occur in older animals.

Beech-nut, Gerber and Heinz, the three major infant-food manufacturers, have discontinued its use in baby foods.

But a few adults have been found to be highly sensitive to large doses of monosodium glutamate. These caused headaches, oppressive feelings (sometimes panic) and gastrointestinal discomfort. This complaint is popularly known as "Chinese restaurant syndrome," because MSG is a common ingredient in Chinese cooking and the effect was first observed in patrons of Chinese restaurants. I personally believe that the use of MSG should be drastically reduced. If you need more flavor, why not select better cooking?

There are said to be certain additives called "improving agents." What are they and what are their functions?

This group includes chemicals such as lecithin for glazing confectionery and improving the shine on bakery products, and enzymes for bettering the taste and consistency of many foods.

The nitrite additives, undergoing a thorough reevaluation in this country, have been found to cause a change in the chemistry of the blood of young experimental animals. The possible risk of cancer from nitrites, claimed by certain scientists, is very iffy and depends on their hypothetical combination with naturally occurring amines. There is no experimental confirmation of this risk, but the use of nitrites is now limited in amounts and in types of foods in which they can be used.

No ill effects have been reported from the presence of enzymes—which are proteins that seem to be digested like other proteins.

Aren't the natural colors of foods satisfactory to food processors? What makes them add dyes to their products?

Dyes are commonly employed because many foods lose their natural color when processed. Pale foods tend to discourage appetite—and customers. As "synthetic" foods replaced the original products, artificial colors were introduced to reinforce taste.

Something that looks the way we expect it to, tastes better to us. Banana ice cream made with artificial banana flavor will not be accepted unless it has the color as well as the flavor of banana.

The restoration of the original color by artificial means can perhaps be justified if it helps the consumption of a useful food, even though none of the dyes used has any nutritional value itself. But the use of arbitrary color in new products can be defended only on purely aesthetic grounds and I believe that many such colors could well be eliminated.

I have just prepared a list from the labels of various items in my pantry and in my refrigerator. Among the ingredients declared to be in things my family and I expect to eat are: sodium alginate, vegetable agaroid, disodium pyrophosphate and magnesium carbonate. What are they doing on our menu?

Jelling agents and stabilizers are put into food products to keep jellies in a gel state and to keep ice cream creamy. Pectin, sodium alginate, agar, and vegetable gums and starches are the agents commonly added to jellies and baby foods. Ice cream stays in the condition we prefer with the addition of such stabilizers as agar, vegetable agaroid, sodium alginate, methylcellulose and sodium caseinate.

Other stabilizers, calcium lactate, calcium chloride, disodium pyrophosphate and sodium triphosphate (all are minerals found in nature), are used to improve a variety of products, such as fish cakes, sausages and instant potato flakes.

Emulsifiers, which prevent oil and water from separating, are added to bakery products and to margarine. Closely related to them are what are known as "plasticizers" and "antispattering agents." Inorganic salts, such as potassium and magnesium

carbonates, and complex organic substances, such as phospha-
tides, are also used.

>*What with all the additives you've mentioned, the hundreds
you haven't and new ones apparently appearing all the time,
is the Food and Drug Administration sufficiently staffed
and funded to keep a useful eye on everything offered us to
eat?*

Obviously the screening of all new compounds should be
thorough. Additional safety standards should be set to cut
down on the proliferation of new compounds, thereby reducing
the chances that another unsafe additive might threaten the
consumer.

Moreover, additives already on the FDA's "Generally
Recognized as Safe" (GRAS) list should be subjected to the
same searching investigation as new compounds and, in fact,
since the 1969 White House Conference on Food, Nutrition
and Health, a serious review of the safety of the GRAS additives has been undertaken. It is perhaps well to point out that
cancer existed millions of years before food additives were invented—and even natural foods probably contain deadly uni-
dentified substances.

Though the FDA has the primary responsibility for ensur-
ing a safe and nutritious food supply, its food-investigating
budget, inadequate in 1960, has been spread even thinner due
to the increased volume of food products.

In 1961 that budget was $11 million. Its 1,059 employees
inspected food plants, tested samples, and carried out the ad-
ministrative tasks of regulating the multibillion-dollar industry.

The FDA's 1974 food safety budget rose to $69.3 million.
This sixfold increase was less than it would initially appear
when we take into account the inflation factor. Still, it was
sizable. Eleven hundred and four new employees were added to
regulate an industry in which the consumer spent $130 billion
in 1974. (It is interesting to note that the FDA's food-safety
budget represented one-half of one-thousandth of the total cost
of food.)

>*What more can be done to give greater protection to con-
sumers of food—that is, everybody?*

The FDA must have the necessary means to do its job. And a unified code for all the states would also help. But, despite the problems, we are eating far more safely than our forebears did. And absolute safety can never be guaranteed.

Is it safe to store the unused portion of canned food in the can after opening it?

Yes, it is. The important thing to remember is to refrigerate it promptly to avoid unnecessary bacterial growth that can cause spoilage.

Certain acid foods, such as orange or grapefruit juice or canned citrus sections, will dissolve a little of the iron from the inside of the can after a period of time. While this is not harmful or dangerous, the metallic taste the iron gives to the food is undesirable. Therefore, acid foods, unless consumed in a short period of time, should be stored in a nonmetallic container.

There's been so much publicity about botulism that I am fearful of eating food from store-bought cans. Is there any way of detecting bad cans in advance—without experiencing dangerous or fatal symptoms?

Botulism is extremely rare in industrially canned foods. During the past forty years, only seven deaths have occurred in the United States following ingestion of food canned by industry. During the same period, over 700 billion cans of food have been bought from stores! Obviously, it is more dangerous to drive to the supermarket than to consume the contents of the can you bought there.

So far as spotting faulty or damaged cans, food inspectors use a picturesque slang for cans to avoid. They call some of them "flippers." These are cans in which one end pops out if the other is pushed. "Springers," on the other hand, are cans the end of which, if pushed, will pop in and, when pressure is released, pop out. You must assume that these cans contain bacteria that produced poisonous gases thus causing the bulging. Throw these cans away, or, better still, bring them to the nearest office of the Food and Drug Administration.

In addition, throw away every can with any of the following: a dent which includes a seam (side or top or bottom); a break; rust spots. Dents and rust spots may have caused (or, in the case of rust spots, may have been caused by) small leaks through which bacteria can invade the food.

Use your nose when examining a suspected can. If the contents smell bad, however slightly, throw the can away. But don't apply the taste-test! You probably will never encounter a bad can, but why not keep the odds all in your favor?

How real is the threat of botulism poisoning? As a home canner, I am concerned about precautions I should take to prevent it.

As I just pointed out, the incidence of botulism poisoning is really quite low, representing a minute fraction of all reported food poisoning in the United States. When an outbreak does occur, however, it can be quite disastrous. In 1970, six outbreaks were reported. They involved thirteen people. Five died. The overwhelming source of infection was home-canned food.

The problem is that botulism organisms, ubiquitous in gardens, are destroyed very easily by heat. Their spores or cocoons, however, are not. In the absence of air, such as in a sealed can or jar, they begin to grow and produce a highly dangerous toxin. Fortunately, they do not survive in a salty solution, in a 50-percent sugar solution, such as one would use in canning fruit, or in a highly acid solution, as in the case of some canned tomatoes, for example.

This narrows considerably the field of potentially dangerous foods. Among the most common home-canned foods which support growth of the botulism organism are low-acid tomatoes, snap beans, corn, asparagus, peas and spinach.

Here are sensible precautions: never use damaged canned food, especially where the top of the container is puffed up, evidence that bacterial gas is being formed. For the home canner, pressure-cooker cooking is regarded as the safest method in order to produce a heat high enough to kill bacterial spores. As a final security measure, home-canned vegetables should be boiled ten minutes before being eaten.

As a kitchen worker in a restaurant, I have been interested in your comments about food poisoning. You've never written about ptomaine poisoning, though. This used to be pretty common, wasn't it? Don't people get ptomaine poisoning any more?

"Ptomaine poisoning" is a misnomer. What have been referred to as ptomaine poisonings are in the vast majority of cases salmonella infections or food poisoning from toxins produced by bacteria.

Ptomaines do exist. They are products of protein that is so decomposed the food is partly liquefied and is offensive to the senses. Since no human, however hungry, would eat the odoriferous, sulfur-containing ptomaines, this type of poisoning is unlikely to occur.

A few years ago, in an attempt to do the nutritionally right thing, we began to eat less fat and to consume a lot more fish. Those scares about mercury contamination now leave me wondering. What should we do?

Mercury poisoning from our food supply is a negligible risk, made even smaller by the careful monitoring done by federal agencies. Current evidence continues to reinforce the merits of a diet lower in fat (with a relative increase in polyunsaturated and a decrease in saturated fats) and low in cholesterol.

You will be doing yourselves and your hearts a good turn by continuing to eat fish frequently. Even shellfish, which contain more cholesterol but are very low in fat, can be included occasionally in your diet.

Our local newspaper ran an article describing an outbreak of gastroenteritis at a large gathering. I was astonished to read that spaghetti and meat sauce was found to be the problem. What is there in spaghetti and meat sauce that would cause diarrhea?

The food-poisoning incident was probably due to the way the spaghetti was handled. This disturbance could have occurred with any number of prepared foods.

Microorganisms, normally present and harmless in small amounts, are allowed to multiply to an extent where they can produce symptoms of food poisoning. This frequently takes place when food for large groups is prepared in deep containers and allowed to cool slowly at room temperature, providing ample time for bacterial growth. The important conclusion for church-supper cooks: once you put a meal together, place it in shallow pans, not more than four inches deep. Stir frequently to hasten thorough cooling of the entire mixture and refrigerate promptly. Never let your beef stew or whatever sit around for hours on a kitchen counter cooling and incubating bacteria.

Is it safe to store spaghetti and meat sauce in the aluminum pot in which it is cooked?

The important point here is not the aluminum pot but how you handle the sauce, as just explained, once it is cooked.

Aluminum pots have been the target of unsubstantiated attacks by critics for many years. Aluminum is the third most common element in the earth's crust, and therefore occurs naturally in many foods. And pickles are kept crunchy by adding alum which, of course, contains aluminum. Minute amounts do dissolve in the ordinary cooking process, especially if the mixture is alkaline, but all the tests which have been done so far have shown that the amount of aluminum ingested from cookware is far less than from other sources and is truly insignificant.

Can you get hepatitis from eating crab, shrimp and scallops, as well as from clams and oysters? And if shellfish containing the hepatitis virus are cooked, can you still get the disease?

The two shellfish which have been identified as a source of the hepatitis virus are clams and oysters. While the minimum cooking period for safety remains unknown, twenty minutes has been found effective in killing the hepatitis agent. But, as any New Englander can tell you, this would make a steamed clam far too tough for you to enjoy.

Prevention of hepatitis from shellfish, therefore, depends on good community sanitation and constant surveillance to insure that shellfish are harvested only from uncontaminated water. In practical terms for the consumer, this means that you must be sure to buy shellfish from a reputable source. It can be hazardous to do your own digging in flats where there is the slightest question regarding the purity of the water.

Some time ago I opened some canned shrimp and noticed something in it which resembled glass. I didn't know what to do so I threw it out. What is this substance, and is it harmful?

What you undoubtedly found is something called struvite, crystals of magnesium ammonium phosphate which occasionally form in canned seafood from normally present constituents. Although this is not attractive, its presence does not affect the safety of the food.

The seafood canning industry has spent considerable effort to try to solve the struvite problem, but to date they have been unsuccessful.

Incidentally, the sure way to distinguish struvite from glass is to place the crystals in warm vinegar. If they are struvite, the crystals will dissolve in a short while.

How much of a danger to our food and, thus, to us is the fallout of radioactive materials from nuclear explosions in the atmosphere? Is it true that something called strontium-90 adds to the threat of cancer?

The most dangerous of the radioactive elements that settle on land and water after a nuclear explosion above the earth's surface, are strontium-90, cesium-137 and iodine-131. In forty days only about 1/32 of the iodine is left. But half of the cesium is still with us after thirty years, half of the strontium after twenty-eight years.

Cesium reaches us and can accumulate in our soft tissues when we eat the meat of animals whose own soft tissues have acquired it when they grazed. Strontium brings about irreparable harm to our bone marrow. It is believed that strontium adds to the threat of bone tumors and of leukemia.

Cows get strontium in grass. We get it in their milk. So, of course, do children, who are most susceptible to damage to their bones.

Authorities are, in the main, not disturbed by this, but the sooner the testing of all nuclear weapons is stopped, and the weapons are effectively banned, the better.

19 LABELING— WHAT'S IN IT FOR YOU?

The final report of the White House Conference on Food, Nutrition and Health in December of 1969 included the recommendation of a distinguished panel that the (food-processing) industry voluntarily "promote the concept of a balanced diet for all citizens through the use of uniform words, symbols or other graphic devices. . . ."

In my letter of transmittal of the report to the President, I complimented industry leaders for their cooperative and forward-looking consideration of the problems involved in packaging and labeling, "including the meaningful description of nutritional information."

In the following month, in an interview in *Psychology Today,* I emphasized that the "Government can, I think, ask the food industry to list the number of calories per serving in each package and maybe indicate the nutrient composition as well so people will know what they're eating."

One year later, writing in *Family Health,* I declared that "our labeling regulations were designed for a simpler era, when most meals were prepared in the home from start to finish. The combination of technological advances and increasing affluence have changed all that, but labeling rules haven't caught up with this food revolution. Clearly, these rules must be updated to meet the needs of the 1970s, so that every housewife will have the information she needs to ensure good nutrition for her family.

"Our lack of information about the contents of processed foods—including anything canned, frozen or packaged—is becoming a real problem. About one-third of all the food we eat today is eaten outside the home, much of it consisting of the highly processed components of sandwiches and other instant meals. Half the food we eat at home is highly processed. Do we know what is in it and what is not?"

It was heartening to me to be able to report that the Food and Drug Administration was working on the final details of a new national policy concerning labeling. And again I seconded the motion.

"Why," I demanded, "make a great effort to provide good nutrition education unless people can apply it by being able to choose the most nutritious foods? . . . We can exhort people to eat polyunsaturated fat until they finally begin to believe it, only to be frustrated when they get to the grocery and look for some."

I suggested, "if the main vitamins, minerals or polyunsaturated fats are listed on the label it might give the food industry greater incentive to increase the proportion of these valuable nutrients in their products.

"The labeling of key nutrients may help insure that in processed foods the needed vitamins and minerals haven't been lost. But the labels will have to make sense. The nutritional listings shouldn't be so detailed that they become incomprehensible. They should give the key nutrients in such a way that they can be easily read and related to familiar measurements. One good possibility is to label each food with the number of calories per common portion, with ratings to indicate how much each portion contributes to the fulfillment of daily requirements of a number of nutrients. The buyer would then know not only what a given food is rich in, as present advertising emphasizes, but what other combinations of foods must be served in order to provide a complete diet.

1   "The FDA has already proposed new regulations along

such lines for infant foods, especially those, such as formulas, that constitute the sole diet of some infants. These products would be required to carry label information about quality or quantity of protein, moisture, carbohydrates, calories, vitamins and minerals. If there is not enough protein to meet nutritional demands, the label would have to say that the product shouldn't be the only source of protein for the infant. Whole cow's milk and evaporated milk would not be affected. But milk offered as a substitute for human milk would have to carry a label saying whether it contained vitamin C and D supplements and additional iron.

"Once the Food and Drug Administration has worked out the details of its overall new policy, it hopes, through cooperation with food chains and food processors, to begin experimenting with labels. In this way, the most effective, informative guides can be worked out. I believe this is essential if our current push toward better nutrition education, a drive supported by government agencies, schools, industries, and private foundations, is to work with any degree of success."

It was not until April of 1972 that I was able to begin a report, again in *Family Health,* with the welcome words, "Nutritional labeling has arrived." And I nodded my appreciation to the first stores to adopt it. They included: the Giant Food Stores in the Washington, D.C., area (which pioneered the use of unit pricing), Jewel Stores, First National, and Kroger. Then I went on to explain how the system worked.

"Here's what the Giant Food labels are now showing: Calories per household portion (by the ounce, the cup, the glass, or whatever the most common measure is). Carbohydrates, protein, and fats, how many grams per portion. Other nutrients rated to show the percentage each portion contributes to the Recommended Daily Allowance of vitamins A, C, B_1, B_2, niacin, iron and calcium. Vitamin D, when added to milk or cereals.

"The nutrient ratings are shown as simple numbers from 0 to 10, with 10 indicating that one portion of the food contains 100 percent of the Recommended Daily Allowance for that vitamin or mineral, 9 meaning 90 percent, and so on down the nutritional scale.

212   "The Jewel Stores' system is similar. The labeling is hon-

est. It shows what is in the food and what is not. By reminding the consumer that no single food contributes all the needed nutrients in ideal amounts, it underscores the need for a varied diet. Finally, this labeling gives a simple guide to follow to achieve the daily allowance for all the main nutrients: the sum of all portions consumed during the day should add to 10 for each of the nutrients listed."

The public reaction to these pilot systems showed that, while shoppers were wholeheartedly in favor of nutritional labeling, they wanted it "straight," i.e., they wanted "100 percent" not by 10; "50 percent" by "50 percent," not by 5 and so on.

The final regulations, introduced in 1973 and now in effect, follow this "percentage" system. The percentages on the new nutrition labels are based on the "U.S.R.D.A." The U.S.R.D.A. have condensed the seventeen categories of requirements in the National Academy of Sciences' *Recommended Dietary Allowances* into four: for infants up to one year old, for children from one to three years, for older children and adults, and for pregnant and lactating women. The requirements are usually the highest values in each category for each nutrient.

These long-awaited regulations on food labeling were presented in three parts:

The first set covers the labeling of processed foods. The label must show the number of calories in an average portion; number of grams of protein; carbohydrate and fat; and the proportion that each serving makes toward your daily needs of particular vitamins and minerals, provided the food contains more than 2 percent of the U.S.R.D.A.

The second set is concerned with the labeling of the type of fat contained in edible fats, oils and shortenings. This labeling tells you the amount of saturated fat, polyunsaturated fat and cholesterol in each of these products.

The third group of regulations establishes standards for vitamins and minerals sold as dietary supplements. And it makes a little sense of the use of the word "imitation." Now the term will have to be shown prominently on foods that are like the real things but less nutritious. It will no longer be required on foods that are just as nutritious.

Up until now, with a few exceptions, all you could learn

from the label on a product was the ingredients in the order of greatest proportion. If the list said, "water, sugar, peaches," it meant more water than sugar, more sugar than peaches. There was no way to know whether there was just a little more water or that the can contained 90 percent water, 8 percent sugar, and 2 percent peaches. Nutritional labeling partly closes this gap as well.

Nutritional labeling, on a large scale, is new and, inevitably, like anything else just becoming familiar, it generates questions:

Is nutritional labeling of particular help to those who are counting calories?

It is essential. Knowledge of the number of calories per portion will dispel some of the old chestnuts (or canards) which have doomed many a dieter's efforts: the belief that meat is all protein; that protein is calorie-free; or that only carbohydrate foods are fattening. Nutritional labeling informs the consumer that bread, in weight and calories, is 13 percent protein while the calories of hamburger may be over 70 percent fat. More generally, the reading of nutritional labels will show that there are no "thinning" foods as opposed to "fattening" foods, and that portion size is an important factor in weight control.

Are there any other values in calorie-content labeling?

It's the only way in which the dieter will be able to use processed and "convenience" foods. Even if one were willing to keep a table of caloric content handy at the store and at the dinner table, such compilations do not contain the calorie count of the new foods, nor would they ever be able to keep up with the seemingly endless variety of modifications marketed by competing firms. There are now thousands of such "complex" foods and only tables as thick as telephone books (with regular supplements to cover the four hundred new foods introduced each month) could cope with the numbers involved.

What can be done to make labels even more informative?

It is to be hoped that sometime in the future the label will tell you at least the percentage of the main ingredient (how much turkey in turkey pie, etc.).

214

The advocates of this type of labeling believe it is most needed because of a Gresham's Law ("bad money drives out good") of the food industry. They ask us to consider conscientious manufacturers A and B, each of whom has a recipe calling for a lot of chunks of turkey meat in their frozen turkey pies. Manufacturer C enters the market with a lavishly advertised frozen turkey pie, encased in a box adorned with a picture of a pie as steaming and succulent as those on the covers of existing pies and appreciably cheaper. Pie C also contains much less turkey. Without obligatory labeling conspicuously revealing the quantity of turkey in turkey pie, manufacturers A and B will be forced to lower the turkey content of their pies if they're going to sell them at a more competitive price. Proper labeling is thus a guarantee to the quality manufacturer that he will get the price to which his product entitles him.

What about the nutrients which are not *on the label?*

You have put your finger on the one real problem of interpreting nutritional labeling. If you are dealing with a lightly processed food—say, canned animal product, fruit or vegetable —adequacy in a number of listed vitamins and minerals usually indicates that the food also provides a number of unlisted nutrients, "secondary" vitamins, such as pyridoxine, folic acid, or vitamin B_{12}, and trace minerals, such as magnesium, copper, or zinc. On the other hand, if you are dealing with a highly refined, "semisynthetic" food which is enriched with a number of listed nutrients, such as an enriched, high-sugar refined cereal, the list only indicates what is on it and nothing else.

Once again, this points out the wisdom of eating a varied diet, made up primarily of unprocessed or lightly processed foods.

Are all these FDA rules mandatory on all packaged products of all manufacturers?

If a food is described as "enriched" or "low in calories" or any claim is made that it is nutritious, the manufacturer must follow the rules—all the rules, not merely those relevant to the particular claim made. They are also mandatory if a given food is purported to constitute a full meal or is presented as an infant or "dietetic" food.

I've been particularly interested in your advocacy of "in-gredient-listing" (the how-much-turkey theme). Why don't you regard it as important to list all the ingredients? There are thousands of people who are allergic to hundreds of foods. Wouldn't a complete answer to the question "What's in it?" protect many of them from major discomfort, serious disease or worse?

I do agree that all ingredients, with the possible exceptions of those known to be harmless in small quantities for everyone should be listed on the package. All of fourteen bills, in one way or another with that end in view, have been introduced in the House of Representatives and been referred to the Interstate and Foreign Commerce Committee. I hope the members of that committee will read thoughtfully a letter written in April 1972 by a Dedham, Massachusetts, father. He wrote:

"My son had an allergy to peanuts all his life . . . the plastic cover of the ice cream did not say anything on it about it containing peanuts. On Monday, ten-year-old Michael passed away from natural causes due to glottic edema [swelling of the tongue] and anaphylatic reaction due to ingested peanuts."

Doesn't the presence of nutrient ratings on the label compli-cate rather than simplify shopping by the already put-upon housewife?

To the contrary. Living with and profiting from the new data is quite simple. It requires no postgraduate course in nutri-tion and statistical analysis. It's an easy matter of choosing several numbers that add up to 100.

I know dozens of housewives who can go into a grocery store, fill a cart to overflowing, and calculate in their heads almost exactly how much it will all cost before they get to the check-out counter.

Not only are women quite capable of understanding the most comprehensive labeling system but they are glad to see the task of building balanced meals made more rational than ever before.

There's dramatic proof in the experience of one company which instituted nutritional labeling in an inner-city area where formal education is presumably as low as income. When the shoppers in that store started reading the nutritional labels at the meat counter, sales of liver boomed. The store couldn't keep up the demand. Apparently, it is one thing to hear nutritionists praise liver as "good for you," but it's quite another thing to see for yourself how favorably it compares with more expensive meats in real terms—just as much protein but only one-fifth the fat and half the calories of steak; twice as much iron per calorie; 1,000 times as much vitamin A per portion and several times as much of the B vitamins.

How does "unit-pricing" fit in with the nutrient ratings now appearing on the labels of so many products?

Unit-pricing continues to provide consumers with a useful weapon in the battle for food bargains. Each food has two prices clearly marked on the shelf where the product is presented. One is the cost of the item and the other is the cost per pound. (In the event, a frequent happening, that the item itself contains 16 ounces, the prices shown are, of course, identical.) One motive for unit-pricing, a self-serving one from which the shopper benefits, is that the "store-brand" is usually the economical buy and the price benefit encourages its sale.

Why aren't the ingredients listed on packaged ice cream? Are the less expensive ones just as good?

Ice cream is one of the foods for which there is a federal "standard of identity" for the specific ingredients and the proportions in which they must occur have been standardized. Only optional ingredients must be listed.

The standard for ice cream states that it must contain not less than 10 percent butterfat. Other ingredients include milk solids, sweeteners (usually cane and corn syrup solids) and a small amount of stabilizers and emulsifiers to insure smoothness.

Coloring may also be added without declaring it on the label, a note of importance to anyone allergic to food coloring.

There may be a number of reasons for cost variation but the major one is butterfat content. While 10 percent is the minimum set by the federal government, the manufacturer is free to add more fat to make it a richer product. This, of course, drives up both cost and calories.

A one-half cup serving of regular ice cream with a 10 percent fat content contains about 125 calories and an amount of fat equal to about 1½ teaspoons of butter. The same portion of rich ice cream, containing 16 percent fat, provides an additional 40 calories and a total of 2½ teaspoons of butterfat.

With current emphasis on a lowered intake of saturated fat and cholesterol, the prudent option is the lower-fat product. And, if you're really interested in reducing fat intake, remember that a half cup of ice milk contains about 100 calories and only a half teaspoon of fat.

I recently read a comment by a food-industry executive who said that consumers are as likely to leave the market with a watered-down orange drink as with 100 percent orange juice and not even know it. I went to the market and took a careful look. I was certainly confused by all the different names. Can you straighten me out?

Being an enlightened orange juice consumer these days is no easy matter. And the controversy over names and categories of juice drinks containing less than 100 percent juice has been going on for years.

Recently, the FDA set up new standards for various orange juice products. You can buy juice drinks which contain between 35 and 69 percent orange juice, orange drink with 10 to 34 percent orange juice, or orange-flavored drink with from 0 to 10 percent orange juice, not to mention frozen concentrates of imitation orange juice.

In comparing the price of pure orange juice with sugar-water-juice combinations, one finds it is quite possible to buy frozen orange juice for the same price (or even less) per serving as an orange drink, which incidentally costs more in glass than in cans.

One reason consumers may be selecting orange drink without even knowing it is the marketing. The label pictures tempting, ripe oranges dripping juice into elegant crystal stemware. But the beauty of the label masks the uninteresting contents. And often the "juice drinks" stand side by side with the true juices. Without a careful look, it is quite simple for the busy shopper to emerge from the store with orange-flavored sugar water!

As the housewife becomes increasingly conscious of the fine print on the orange drink label, however, she will be less and less likely to buy sugar water when, for the same money, she can get pure orange juice.

20 SOME PRACTICALITIES: BUYING FOOD

The next time you're in a supermarket wondering whether you'd get the best nutrition from a well-trimmed head of fresh lettuce, a package of frozen corn, or a can of beets, take my advice. Buy all three.

Better still, look around the produce section for lettuce that has a lot of leaves and try to get one that was grown nearby, not shipped across country. When you open the can of beets, don't pour the juice down the drain; use it to make borscht. Plan to serve the frozen corn the week you buy it, and keep it solidly frozen until the minute you put it in the pot.

Since you're not likely to have a professional nutritionist along with you on many shopping trips, let us explore some questions about this whole process of shopping:

How can I apply the specific advice you just gave to the selection of all sorts of other foods?

It's easy, once you know the reasoning behind my recommendations. For instance, there isn't any one solution to the problem: "Which is the best, canned, fresh or frozen?" Each in its own way and its own season has its drawbacks and its values. And since it is practically impossible to pick each food for its specific nutritional value—even with the recent improvements in labeling—the best way to ensure proper nutrition is to use all kinds of produce in profusion and variety. Then, use each to its best advantage by careful handling and cooking.

Start with two basic facts:

First, nutrition can be lost (though sometimes even gained) by heat, water, trimming, shipping, storing and thawing.

Second, changes in nutrition can be so subtle or so complex that it's hard even for a scientist to know what he's getting out of what he's eating.

Can I not safely assume that fresh fruits and vegetables must be more nutritious than anything processed?

For the most part, you're on firm ground. But when "fresh" produce is harvested in California and shipped by train or truck to the East Coast, the days spent in transit inevitably result in loss of nutrients.

Not only that, but the vegetables, and particularly the fruit, selected to survive this long journey generally have to be plucked before they are completely ready and thus reach their destination in an imperfect state of ripeness.

Then there's the matter of season. Much as you might enjoy a juicy peach in mid-December, I doubt whether peaches from Chile, not very ripe when picked and probably long-traveled, are much of a nutritional bargain. (They're certainly not a financial one.)

And some produce, of course, simply isn't available from *anywhere* in the off season. Fresh, locally grown, picked-when-ripe-and-rushed-to-market produce is indeed superior in season. But the variety of processed foods available out of season are invaluable in filling the gaps. And they are convenient.

Whether it's fresh food or processed, what effect does trimming have on the nutritional value?

Trimming diminishes it somewhat. There's more vitamin C, for example, in the peel and just under the skin of apples, tomatoes and citrus fruit than on the inside. Inner leaves of cabbage, lettuce and similar vegetables are practically devoid of carotene, but the outer green leaves are loaded with it. You lose a little niacin when you peel carrots, a little riboflavin when you peel a potato.

Since slicing and dicing expose some vitamins to air, where the oxygen partly destroys them, whole fruits and vegetables (either fresh or processed) are generally more nutritious than bits and pieces of such foods.

Does the canning process bring about any loss in nutrition?
Yes, there is some limited loss, mostly occurring in blanching, a step common to both canning and freezing.

The first step in both processes is thorough cleaning of the food by high-pressure sprays or strong-flowing streams of clean water as the food moves on a belt or on revolving screens. Next comes the blanch, immersion in hot water or exposure to live steam.

Although this is where some vitamins get lost, the blanching is essential, for it makes the product shrink and become firmer and expels residual gases, thus permitting proper filling of the container. Equally important, blanching stops any further action by the enzymes naturally present in the fruit or vegetable. If it weren't for this, the fruit would "digest" itself, produce gas, or soften, wilt and discolor.

After blanching, what happens to canned and frozen foods?
At this point, they go their separate ways. Canned foods, raw and without lids, just pass through an exhaust box in which hot water or steam expands the food and gets rid of air or other gases.

Then the can is immediately sealed hermetically, heat-processed, and cooled. During the cooling, water vapor condenses in the head space of the can and the heated contents contract, which creates the partial vacuum normally present in canned foods. Sometimes, high vacuum is also applied to the can while it's being sealed, thus the term "vacuum packed."

Frozen fruits and vegetables, on the other hand, move directly to the flash freezer after the cleaning and blanching. Certain fruits, however, aren't blanched, but instead are packed with sugar syrup and ascorbic acid or some other oxygen-fighter to prevent loss of vitamins and color.

What particular harm does heat do to foods?
Several vitamins are destroyed by heat, most importantly vitamin C. Others are not only destroyed by heat but they also

leak out in the cooking water. Vitamin B_1 is one of these easily lost vitamins.

Vitamin A and carotene (which the body converts to vitamin A) are heat-resistant and aren't lost in processing. Riboflavin and niacin are heat-resistant but do dissolve in the water. The most recent research shows that blanching eliminates a large proportion of vitamin B_6, pantothenic acid, biotin and folic acid. This can be critical, because these B vitamins aren't put back into foods by enrichment, as are vitamins B_1, B_2 and niacin in flour, bread and breakfast cereal.

There are also some important differences in what happens to the vitamins in various products. Spinach, which is very sensitive, for instance, loses most of its vitamin C when processed.

Many vitamins, of course, aren't *lost* in processing. They simply come out in the cooking water and are still in the can when you drain the liquid in the sink. You'd be much better off using it for something, boiled down for a sauce, put in the blender with fresh vegetables for a vegetable cocktail or added to the grand old standby, soup.

What untoward effects do storage and packaging have on foods?

Canned foods lose nutrients very slowly by staying on the shelf, so it's always a good idea to use things fairly rapidly. The greatest loss usually is the vitamin C in canned juices, but even so you shouldn't lose more than 20 percent in two years. I don't think many housewives keep canned juice that long.

Release of nutrients from stored frozen foods depends mostly on temperature. At zero degrees Fahrenheit not even sensitive vitamin C gets lost easily. But at 32 degrees Fahrenheit, you may deplete vitamin C appreciably over a course of weeks, somewhat less for others. Consequently, to avoid any prolonged periods of warmth, put frozen vegetables into the pot straight from the freezer. Frozen foods served without cooking should be eaten as soon as defrosted.

Packaging makes a difference, too. Although containers have been much improved, tin cans still protect vitamin C values better than paper even if it is impregnated with wax. Foil also keeps out more oxygen than paper, thus helping to preserve nutrients.

Am I supposed to remember which foods have what percentage of which nutrients left in them after processing and packaging?

If you're beginning to lose track, you're not alone. Nutritionists have the same trouble. For example, according to one study, asparagus keeps a lot of vitamins when it's processed, close to 100 percent of vitamin C, niacin, riboflavin and thiamine. Lima beans don't keep as much of any of these and they lose more of one vitamin than another. Not only that, but the amount of vitamins retained after processing varies from one company to another by as much as 40 to 50 percent.

The matter of vitamin B$_6$ is typical. It is not one of the vitamins that are added to enriched foods. Professor Henry Schroeder, a Dartmouth Medical School physician widely known for his studies of trace elements in nutrition, completed studies of the effect of processing on B$_6$ and on certain other vitamins and minerals.

He found that the loss due to canning is over 60 percent for roots, over 75 percent for legumes, over 50 percent for green vegetables and over 35 percent for fruit and fruit juices. While his figures are disputed by some as too high, there is little doubt there are losses and that they depend on the type of food and process used.

Freezing seems to be a somewhat better operation when it comes to the particular vitamins and minerals he studied, but the losses are still substantial. Frozen fruit and fruit juices seem to survive best of all in processing, probably because they are not blanched. But just to complicate matters, for instance, Professor Schroeder also found that weight for weight, canned beets actually gained in manganese and in zinc, compared to fresh raw beets. Presumably this is because these minerals are retained in the pulp and what is lost in processing is the juice, which is poor in these particular minerals.

If remembering all these data is impossible for laymen and women and scientists alike, can nothing be done to assure getting the right vitamins and minerals in the right quantities and in the proper mix?

Few people obviously can attempt to do their shopping on a "specific vitamin" basis, that is, trying to buy one food for vitamin A and another for C and so on, unless all labels are clearly marked for major vitamin content. Nor, if you live in the northern part of the country, can you get all your nutrition from a straight diet of fresh, locally grown foods. The winter is too long and too barren. The best safety, in nutrition as in some other things, is in numbers: try to consume a number of fruits and vegetables of all kinds.

One more thing to keep in mind: If you're anxious to get the most nutrition for the fewest calories, be wary. One brand of "straight" frozen asparagus cuts and tips contains only 25 calories per half-cup portion. The same company's frozen asparagus cuts and tips "in hollandaise sauce" contain 84. Another company's "French-style frozen green beans" contain 26 calories per portion, but when "frozen in butter sauce," the count rises to 63 calories. "Brown-sugar-glazed" carrots contain 114 calories per portion compared to 42 calories for carrots "in butter sauce."

Then there's the final problem: what about the syrup? Some of the nutrients in fruit come out in the stewing juice. If you pour out the syrup, you lose the nutrients, although you also dispense with a lot of sugary calories. If calories don't matter, then by all means enjoy the juice, too, but at least make it "light" syrup, not "heavy."

If weight does weigh on your mind and dental health gnaws at your conscience, then pour out the juice, but be sure you get those vitamins somewhere else. It's the same basic principle we applied to the problem of canned, fresh or frozen. It isn't possible to win with only one card. Deal yourself a winning combination instead.

Every time I go to the supermarket it seems there are new convenience foods available. How can one evaluate their nutritional benefits and relative costs over dishes you can make in your own kitchen?

Evaluating processed foods requires examining products one by one and comparing them—for taste acceptability, cost, and, of course, nutritional benefit—with their homemade counterparts.

For example, an inexpensive chicken pie with only one-half as much chicken as the one you prepare at home is hardly the same product. The government has published some findings on convenience foods. They found that a beef TV dinner costs 25 percent more than a homemade meal; a TV fried chicken dinner costs twice as much as one you prepare yourself. Beef pies also cost twice as much as homemade. Frozen chow mein costs up to 80 percent more.

Convenience main dishes can be particularly valuable to a busy housewife when time is a factor. For someone living at home alone, convenience main dishes provide greater variety with minimum effort or cooking equipment. But one word of caution: serving sizes tend to be small and those who use them regularly must augment them with whole-grain or enriched bread, fresh fruit and milk or skim milk.

I shop once a week and always buy cold cuts for family lunches. At the end of the week, I usually have some left over. My husband says I should throw them out. I think they're still good. Which of us is right?

I agree with you, but with some qualification. One of the major, often unknown, factors is the length of time the cold cuts have been in the store. Some sliced, packaged cold cuts carry dates, although as yet there are no government standards and little uniformity.

The package date may indicate when the food was actually packaged, or it can be the last day a store may sell the product, allowing the consumer a reasonable time for use. Or it can be the so-called quality assurance date, meaning that until the date shown, the product will be of the same quality as when it left the processing plant. Most mysterious of all is a coded date which, once deciphered, can carry such information as production date and last day of sale or shelf life. The only way to know the type of dating, if any, your store is using is to ask the manager.

You may find that a code book has been unobtrusively hanging by the delicatessen case virtually untouched for months. You might also want to consider buying cold cuts sliced to order from the loaf. Many large markets operate a

226

delicatessen counter where the same brand available in packages is offered in bulk. Sometimes the bulk price is less per pound. Besides, that way you can buy exactly as much as you need, avoiding the leftover problem.

I am enclosing a label from a single-serving gelatin type dessert. You'll note that the label states it contains water, sugar, some additives, flavoring and coloring. Is there any food value in this or is it, like soft drinks, just some calories?

Your assessment that it is quite like a soft drink is astutely accurate. You might be interested to know that some supermarket research showed that this single serving of dessert in a can cost about six times as much as a serving of gelatin prepared from a package.

The single-serving puddings, such as vanilla or chocolate, do a little better both nutritionally and in terms of cost. Most contain some skim milk. But they cost about twice as much as a serving of pudding prepared at home with a pudding mix and some powdered milk. As a nutrition-conscious and cost-aware consumer, you'll want to choose desserts carefully and return to the good, old-fashioned, do-it-yourself method.

In the past few months I've noticed a new type of cream with a very long keeping quality is on the market. Is it nutritionally different from regular table cream?

No. It is the same product exposed to a new technologic process. Regular cream is pasteurized by heating to 165 degrees F. for 15 to 18 seconds. The new type of cream, called different things by different manufacturers, is "superpasteurized." That is, it is heated to 290 degrees F. for a fraction of a second. This destroys not only the live bacteria, but nearly all the spores as well. It is then a practically sterilized product packaged in a specially sanitized container.

While in the supermarket the other day, I spent a few minutes browsing among the various powdered drinks and liquid supplements. They seemed to be in two sections of the store, one with the diet foods, the other—specifically the instant breakfasts—with the cereals. With so much variety to choose from and so much information on the cans and packages, I was baffled as to which to choose, or whether I should choose any at all.

I understand your confusion. It is certainly a commentary on the wonders of product development and Madison Avenue marketing that a food as unglamorous and difficult to promote as nonfat dry milk has become the basis for so many popular products.

In the diet food section there are a number of brands for dieters. These average between 175 and 250 calories a serving, depending largely on whether you buy the liquid in a can or reconstitute it yourself with whole or skim milk.

Then, there is a variety sold for those who may need some extra calories. These contain about 375 calories a can. If you look closely, you'll notice that one reason for the greater caloric content is the larger size of the can.

And, finally, there are the instant breakfasts. These vary between 210 and 300 calories, again depending on how they are reconstituted.

The basic ingredients of these products are powdered milk, sugar, flavoring, a bit of preservative, a dash of vitamins and minerals. And the cost is at least two to three times that of a milkshake you could concoct on your own with the ingredients I mention.

These products are perfectly adequate foods, but their merits are no greater than those of the individual ingredients. If you enjoy them and can afford them, by all means continue to drink them. I would not advise you, however, to use them to replace more than one meal a day.

My husband and I are allowed no raw fruits and vegetables. Since I was concerned about the nutrients we may be missing, I considered getting a vegetable juice extractor. After reading about vegetable juice drinks, I became skeptical. What are we missing by not eating raw fruits and vegetables?

If your diet includes a variety of cooked fruits and vegetables, all you're really missing is the roughage which apparently your doctor told you you shouldn't have anyway.

Juicing your own fruits and vegetables can be a pretty

228

expensive way to obtain minerals and vitamins. The juice from a head of lettuce costing in 1974 between 39¢ and 59¢ (depending on the season) would supply about 15 percent of a day's vitamin A requirement. Half a cup of frozen mashed squash, which costs about 12¢, supplies about 85 percent.

It would take two heads of lettuce costing a total of 78¢ to $1.18 to get the amount of vitamin C contained in about 6¢ worth of orange juice.

The iron content in the juice of a head of lettuce is about as much as a half-cup serving of spinach, which costs as little as a seventh as much.

Home juicing, obviously, is not cheap.

What are the differences between the various milks available in the market?
The choices in the supermarket milk cooler can be confusing. Milks vary from whole milk, containing 3.5 percent fat and 160 calories a cup, to skim milk with about 0.1 percent fat and 90 calories per cup. Some skim milk is fortified with nonfat dry milk solids, raising the protein and the calorie count. The wise consumer will look for skim milk which is also fortified with vitamins A and D.

In between whole milk and skim milk are a variety of products easily recognized by their advertising agency names, designed to project an image of a youthful, slender you. They are often called 1 percent or 2 percent milks. This refers to the amount of fat they contain. But, buyer, beware!

The composition of these milks, which are made from whole milk, skim milk and nonfat milk solids, varies greatly. The fat content ranges from 0.6 percent to 2.25 percent. The calories can range from about 110 to 135 per cup and it is often impossible to get the calorie content by reading the label.

If you are concerned about the brand of milk you use, your own milk company can provide you with specific product information.

What is the difference between brown rice and white rice?
In general, very little, as long as the white rice is enriched. Brown rice is the whole grain, with just the husk removed, while white rice has the bran removed also. Both contain ap-

proximately 180 calories per cup, chiefly from carbohydrate, and a small amount of calcium, some iron and B vitamins. White rice does contain less magnesium and phosphorous but, as long as rice is not a large fraction of your diet, this is not significant since both minerals are present in a wide variety of foods.

Brown rice has enjoyed an increasing popularity with advocates of the "natural foods" movement. It does have a particular flavor, a somewhat nutlike taste, that many people enjoy. However, it takes almost twice as long to cook as regular white rice, so if you're going to try it, you'd better start supper preparations a bit early. Brown rice does contribute a small amount of bran. A more dependable source is whole-grain bread or "bran" breakfast cereals.

With the high price of fresh fruit, we have been using mostly the canned varieties. Are we losing many of the vitamins by so doing?

No. Canned pears, pineapples and apple sauce compare quite favorably with fresh varieties. In fact, we have seen already that it is even possible that canned products may contain larger amounts of vitamins in some instances. This is because canners are able to pick ripened fruit and preserve it quickly by modern processing methods designed to minimize nutrient losses.

Fruit that is out of season and must be stored and shipped long distances does not profit from the trip. It can lose vitamins en route to the consumer. Unlike the proverbial "good red wine," a good piece of fruit does not improve with age.

What is the difference between ice cream, ice milk and sherbet? And where do the soft frozen dairy desserts fit into the picture?

As far as calories are concerned, there is not really too much difference between ice cream, ice milk and sherbet. Ice milk has about 40 fewer calories per serving than the other two products. However, the composition of the three is somewhat different. Ice cream has the highest fat content, followed by ice milk. Sherbet has the least.

230   Where do the extra calories come from then? Ice milk has

nonfat dry milk solids added, giving it a higher protein content and boosting the calories. Sherbet, on the other hand, contains more sugar.

Most of the soft-serve frozen desserts are ice milk. They contain approximately 140 calories in a serving or 40 fewer than in a serving of ice cream. They contain only about half as much fat as ice cream, but substantially more than sherbet.

What's the best kind of flour?

There are so many kinds of flour, let's just talk about the three most popular. In order of good nutrition, they are: stone-ground; unbleached and enriched; and enriched white.

Many people think that plain unenriched, unbleached white flour is better than enriched white. It isn't, though again, whole grain flour is.

Incidentally, there's a problem with stoneground flour. It should be kept in the refrigerator because the milling process doesn't take out the oils. As a result, the flour may become rancid at room temperature. And this is one reason white flour was invented.

In these days of rising meat prices, we have begun to use a meat tenderizer and are concerned about its safety. What is your advice?

Meat tenderizers (not to be confused with MSG, the flavor enhancer) contain natural enzymes from pineapples or papayas as the active ingredient. Called bromelain or papain, these enzymes are readily destroyed by the heat used to cook the meat. Moreover, any small amount which might remain after cooking is destroyed by the gastric juice in the stomach.

Papain and bromelain are on the GRAS (Generally Recognized as Safe) List of the FDA for use on foods which are to be cooked. A little meat tenderizer on a less expensive but leaner cut of meat not only performs a service to your pocketbook but also to your heart and blood vessels which, of course, can do with less fat than most of us consume.

I've been regularly buying the same brand of apple juice at a store that advertised it as at a "five-cents-off bargain price." The other day I went to another store and found the same product for two cents less than the so-called bargain. What with all the attention the new consumer movement is directing at abuses in the food department, is there any way to make sure that a "bargain" is truly a bargain?

Not where it affects competition and free enterprise.

There is, however, a ruling made by the FDA and the Federal Trade Commission on what are known as "cents-off promotions." The regulations, as stated by the two governmental agencies, define the length and frequency of promotional sales. For example, a product must have been recently sold at the customary price. Moreover, there must be at least a thirty-day lapse between promotional sales; they may not occur more than three times a year and bargain prices cannot be used for more than six months a year for any single size of a commodity.

While these regulations may seem fairly liberal, they are an important step toward ending perpetual promotions based on regular prices. And you, of course, can do in general what you have done already in particular. Shop around now and then. Compare what you're paying for "bargains" to what other people are being charged in other stores.

Why is "buttermilk" so called? My caloric chart shows that it contains only about 85 calories per cup, about the same as skim milk. Also, how does buttermilk compare nutritionally to regular or skim milk?

Originally, buttermilk was the leftover liquid in the churn after the butter was removed. But, nowadays buttermilk is made by adding a specific type of bacteria (streptococcus lactic) to milk which is then incubated at a carefully controlled temperature until the right acidity is reached. Since most buttermilk sold in this country is made from skim milk it is nutritionally equivalent to it.

The continuous rise in meat prices has forced me to pull the reins on the growing food budget a little tighter. I still want to do the best thing for my family, however. Are sources of protein, other than red meat, really as good?

Indeed they are. The protein of fish, poultry, eggs and **232** cheese are as satisfactory for the growth of your children as red meat (and poultry and fish are lower in fat, a plus in a man's diet).

A recent shopping study came up with some interesting information about the cost of animal protein. The least expensive was canned tuna. This was followed by beef liver, cheddar cheese, broiler chickens, turkeys, eggs, liverwurst and ground beef. In that study, it was shown that it cost roughly three times as much to get the same amount of protein from round steak as from tuna. So, by all means, look to the less expensive sources of protein.

Include also dried beans occasionally. Why not a lentil casserole tonight? By using more tuna, as well as other fish, and more poultry in place of red meat, you will be doing your family the additional favor of serving them a diet lower in fat and calories. Again, let me point out that when I say less or least expensive, I am speaking only by comparison with meat. I am all too well aware that the less costly foods have actually gone up faster since 1972 than the more luxurious foods. The relative order of prices, however, has remained roughly the same.

And one last word. When you do buy meat, select lean meat. There are three good reasons: lower fat, fewer calories, and less waste, meaning more servings per pound.

Can you give me information about which canned soups are good sources of protein and other nutrients?

In general, canned soups are not really nutritional powerhouses, although they can provide some protein, calories, minerals and vitamins.

The average serving of only a few canned soups contains as much protein as you normally get in an ounce of meat. These include bean soup with bacon, or bean with smoked pork, cream of chicken, pepper pot, split pea, and beef or vegetable beef. Other soups such as green pea, black bean, cream of asparagus, cream of mushroom and chicken gumbo contain nearly as much. The rest, even when diluted with milk, generally have only a little more protein than a half ounce of meat.

But this does not mean that soup cannot be considered a regular part of lunchtime fare. When you serve canned soups include some other good sources of protein, either as finger foods or in sandwiches. By using leftovers, you can always add to the soup extra amounts of chicken, meat or fish or fresh garden vegetables.

I hear about a new cereal grain called triticale. Can you tell me something about it?

Triticale, a hybrid cereal produced by cross-breeding wheat and rye, is not really new. It was developed in Europe in the late 1800s, but until recently had been grown only on small experimental plots. It is now being produced commercially in the United States, although many technological problems, particularly increasing the yield to that of wheat, remain.

The importance of triticale rests on recent evidence that certain varieties have a higher protein content and amino acid balance than wheat and therefore provide protein of better value for man. To date, triticale flour has been used successfully in pasta and breads and hard rolls, which have a characteristic mild rye flavor.

How do bologna and frankfurters stack up against tuna fish or hamburger as inexpensive sources of protein?

Approximately one-third of the day's protein requirement can be met with a three-ounce serving of tuna or hamburger. To obtain the same amount of protein from bologna, one would have to eat approximately twice as much at more than twice the cost. Three and a half frankfurters, certainly more than the average serving, would supply the same amount of protein at a cost of 50 percent more.

Bacon, by the way, although often regarded as "meat," scores worst of all. It would take ten slices costing two and one half times as much to supply an equal amount of protein.

The least expensive source of protein is dried beans which for approximately 6 cents provide as much protein as an ounce of the most inexpensive cheese at two to three times the cost. You might rightfully argue that the protein quality of cheese is superior to that of beans. However, bean protein can be substantially improved by simply adding some cheese to the casserole. You may achieve the same result with hamburger or

234 leftover meat.

I recently heard about a new type of beef that is being produced with greater amounts of polyunsaturated fats. Is there really such a thing and is it available in this country?

A group of Australian researchers has found a method of raising cattle and sheep on diets supplemented with a specially treated polyunsaturated oil. These animals produced milk and meat with a much higher than usual ratio of polyunsaturated to saturated fat.

The results of a small study in which the researchers themselves ate the meat and dairy products from these animals showed an average drop in blood cholesterol of 10 percent in a three- to four-week period. This effect was observed even though the amount of cholesterol itself in the tested products was the same as that from ordinary animals.

One company in the United States is currently using the Australian feeding process. While the idea offers exciting possibilities for Americans who find it difficult to eat less meat even in the interest of lower blood cholesterol, the availability of polyunsaturated meat and dairy products at your local supermarket remains in the future. And there is already some concern about what the cost of these foods will be.

For the foreseeable future, more fish and chicken, and less beef, lamb and pork, will remain the bywords of the prudent shopper.

Can you explain the difference between pasteurized processed cheese, process cheese food and process cheese spread? Are they all of the same nutritional value?

Pasteurized process cheese, such as the popular American cheese, is made by grinding and mixing natural cheeses, then melting them and adding an emulsifier, as well as some liquid, salt, acid, color and flavorings.

Process cheese food is also a blend of cheeses. It contains less cheese and fat and more milk or whey solids and water.

Process cheese spread closely resembles cheese food, except that it contains still more moisture, less milk fat, and a stabilizer.

Process cheese spread, which contains the most moisture, costs the least, followed by process cheese food. Most expensive is process cheese which contains the most protein per ounce, 15 percent more than cheese food, and 30 percent more than cheese spread.

An ounce of process cheese contains 105 calories, compared to 90 for cheese food and 80 for cheese spread. However, if you eat enough process cheese food or spread to get the same amount of protein as in an ounce of process cheese, you will take in about the same number of calories and the cost will be roughly the same.

I am interested in learning the comparative amounts of fat and cholesterol in the various types of cottage cheese. Is all cottage cheese low in fat and cholesterol or is it only the cottage cheese made with skim milk?

Low-fat and uncreamed cottage cheese are lower in fat and cholesterol than the creamed variety. But even creamed cottage cheese rates extremely well when viewed within the grand scheme of cheeses. Here are some facts:

Uncreamed and low-fat creamed cottage cheese contain only about 2 milligrams of cholesterol per ounce and negligible amounts of fat. Creamed cottage cheese contains about 4 mg. of cholesterol per ounce and about a gram of fat. (That's equal to about a fifth of a teaspoon of butter.) An ounce of cheddar, on the other hand, contains over 30 mg. of cholesterol and more than 9 grams of fat.

It's obvious that cottage cheese in any form is a good low-fat choice.

I'm really confused about the margarines. It seems that they all contain some partially hydrogenated oil. Didn't you say to buy only the ones which contain polyunsaturated oil?

All margarines must contain some hydrogenated fat or else they would be too liquid to spread. The important thing is that the first ingredient listed be a liquid oil, such as corn, cottonseed, soybean or safflower. Avoid those margarines whose first-listed ingredient is either a partially hydrogenated oil or liquid coconut oil which is naturally highly saturated.

Remember, there are acceptable and nonacceptable margarines in both the stick and tub forms, and some manufacturers change the composition of their margarines from time to time. Therefore, read the labels carefully and check them often.

I am always worried about how much fat we are getting in hamburger. Are there any standards or laws governing how much fat can be included in ground meat?

Hamburger, by law, must contain no more than 30 percent fat. This is quite a substantial amount of fat, however. In fact, it's the same as the legal limit for hot dogs.

Strangely enough, we were told until recently there existed no standard method for combining fat and lean to produce hamburger with consistent, predictable percentages of fat. One problem often cited was the variable fat content of the flesh from one animal to another. A further technological problem was the lack of standard methods for determining the fat content of meat.

A group of experts organized by the National Association of Meat Purveyors has been working on this very problem.

A number of supermarkets have started selling various categories of hamburger: "regular," "lean," "extra lean" and "diet." How then can you, the consumer, be sure you're getting what you're paying for? At present, you must largely rely on your butcher to do an honest job, particularly if your store does not categorize the fat content of hamburgers.

On your own, you can also do a couple of things. For example, buy a pound of ground round from two different markets. Broil each under the same conditions. Then measure the fat at the bottom of the pan. Do the test a couple of times. The amounts of fat should be roughly the same.

For a second test, also buy a pound of ground chuck and a pound of ground round at the same market. Again, broil and measure the fat. If you're paying for lean or extra lean meat, you should have less fat in the bottom of the pan.

If butter or oil becomes rancid, is its nutritional value affected?

Yes. When fats become rancid, both vitamin A and vitamin D may be in part destroyed. Fats and oils should be kept in dark containers (hence the fact that some oils come in brown bottles) or at least in a dark place and they should be kept cool. Butter and margarine, of course, belong in the refrigerator.

In order to forestall the oxidative process which causes fats to become rancid, manufacturers add substances called "antioxidants" to a variety of foods. These include margarine, hydrogenated fats, potato chips and peanut butter. And here, at last, is a use for vitamin E. The antioxidant properties of vitamin E, or tocopherol, have long been recognized as a naturally occurring phenomenon in fats.

Tocopherols have been and still are used as additives to retard the spoilage of fats, but they are often replaced by less expensive, commercially manufactured products.

21 MORE PRACTICALITIES: PREPARING FOOD

Good nutrition is not a matter of emphasizing the actual or supposed importance of one or more particular foods. Nor is it a pattern of eating whatever you please or whatever is put before you. The way to keep yourself properly nourished is to accustom yourself to a diet of great variety.

When you do this, you reap some bonuses: The greater the diversity of the foods you eat the lesser the chances you will miss any nutrients and the less the likelihood your meals will become dull. And, more often than not, you'll spend your food dollar with the greatest possible economy.

Planning a varied diet is eased for you by the classification of foods into the "Basic Seven" groups. If you are in good health and if your physician or dietitian has not outlawed a specific food for some sound reason, then each day you should eat at least one serving from every one of the seven groups. Children, depending on age and activity, will need less than a serving. Teen-agers and men and women working vigorously will need more. The Basic Seven food groups are:

(1) leafy, green and yellow vegetables
(2) citrus fruits, tomatoes, raw cabbage, and salad greens
(3) potatoes and other vegetables and fruits

(4) milk and milk products

(5) meat, poultry, fish, eggs, dried beans and peas, and nuts

(6) bread, flour and cereals

(7) butter, fortified margarine and polyunsaturated oils and margarines.

And now, a look at these groups in greater detail.

Group One: Leafy, Green and Yellow Vegetables. Included are carrots, squash, pumpkins, sweet potatoes, wax beans, rutabagas and every kind of green except salad greens, which are classified in a separate group. Group One vegetables may be eaten raw, cooked, canned or frozen. They provide large amounts of vitamin A and many supply iron, calcium, thiamine, riboflavin and vitamin E. What's more, they furnish fiber to help regulate the intestine.

Group Two: Citrus Fruits, Tomatoes, Raw Cabbage, and Salad Greens. Included are not only oranges, lemons, limes and grapefruit but also their juices and fresh berries, too. This group furnishes good sources of vitamins A and C, calcium and iron.

Group Three: Potatoes and Other Vegetables and Noncitrus Fruits. Included are beets, onions, celery, eggplant, corn, parsnips, cucumbers and white turnips. Potatoes, baked or boiled, provide vitamin C. At least one potato a day is suggested for active children and adults. A daily serving of another food from Group Three is also recommended. Fruits in this group include apples, grapes, peaches, pears, pineapples, figs, prunes, raisins, plums and bananas. This group supplies many of the carbohydrates needed by the body, and is a source of vitamins and minerals.

Group Four: Milk and Milk Products. Milk in any form belongs in this group: fresh, dried, evaporated, condensed or made into cheese or ice cream or ice milk. A child should have three or four cups of milk a day, and a grownup at least two cups. Milk and cheese serve as valuable sources of calcium, vitamin A, riboflavin and high-quality proteins. Cheese can be substituted for milk by an adult consuming an otherwise varied diet if he does not like or can't tolerate milk. (Many black and Asiatic adults do not tolerate milk well.) Skim milk is preferable to whole milk for those who have to cut down on calories and saturated fats.

Group Five: Meat, Poultry, Fish, Eggs, Dried Beans and

Peas, and Nuts. The chief source of protein in the diet, as well as a source of energy from the protein and the fat. It provides also vitamin B_1, iron, phosphorus, thiamine and niacin. Dried beans and peas and nuts furnish some starch. One or two servings a day are recommended from among the following:

Meat and poultry of all kinds, including liver, and kidneys, heart and other variety meats.

Fish, fresh, frozen, dried or canned.

Eggs are an excellent source of a variety of nutrients. (Because they are high in cholesterol, associated with heart attacks, they are not recommended for adult men.)

Dried beans and peas, and nuts, including soybeans and peanut butter. When legumes or nuts are substituted for other foods in this group, milk or cheese should be added to supply essential amino acids.

Group Six: Bread, Flour and Cereals. Included are rolls, biscuits and crackers. All of these should be made of wholegrain or enriched flour or cereal because when flours and cereals are milled, much of the outer coat (rich in minerals and vitamins) of the grain is removed. Foods in this group are valuable energy sources and also provide protein.

Group Seven: Butter and Fortified Margarine. Margarine must be fortified with vitamin A to equal the amount normally found in butter. These foods are chiefly energy producers and vitamin A sources. One or the other should be included in the daily diet.

No specific amount is suggested, but their consumption should be limited for persons watching their weight and for adult men who must avoid excessive amounts of saturated fat.

Polyunsaturated oils, though not good sources of vitamin A (except for red palm oil, consumed in certain areas of Africa), also contribute "essential" fatty acids to the diet. Generally, diets for the lowering of blood cholesterol include lowering total calories if the person is overweight, lowering of total fat and replacement of part of the saturated fat by polyunsaturated margarines or oils. If oils replace butter or fortified margarines, care must be taken that sufficient sources of vitamin A remain in the diet. Polyunsaturated margarines are usually fortified with vitamins A and D.

I've checked the freezer compartment of my refrigerator and it stays at about 5°. Can you tell me how long I can safely store meat at that temperature?

This depends on the type of meat and the size of the piece. In general, beef roasts and steaks can be kept up to twelve months and veal or lamb roasts nine months. Pork roasts, however, should be kept no longer than six months. Chops and cutlets should be stored about half as long as roasts, and ground meat and stew only about three months. Chicken, either whole or cut up, will remain in good condition about ten months. While meats kept longer than this are not harmful to eat, the quality does begin to deteriorate.

These storage times assume that the meats are carefully wrapped in moisture- and vapor-proof packaging, such as heavy-duty foil, plastic freezer bags, or other freezer wraps. Meats frozen only in supermarket packaging should be kept no longer than two weeks.

Incidentally, 5° is really the upper temperature limit for long-term storage of frozen food. Authorities generally recommend zero or below. At higher temperatures, food deteriorates far more rapidly.

My husband is Italian and does a lot of the cooking. He insists on using substantial amounts of olive oil in cooking and on salads. Olive oil is considered a neutral oil. Does this mean it is neither harmful nor beneficial?

In scientific terms it means it contains a high proportion of mono-unsaturated fats which are neutral together with some polyunsaturated and saturated fatty acids. The so-called neutral oils are not highly polyunsaturated, as are the corn, cottonseed and soybean oils which are an important part of a cholesterol-lowering diet.

I appreciate your husband's reluctance to eliminate olive oil with its definite flavor. He probably has used it all his life. Here are a few compromises he can make:

Switch to one of the polyunsaturated oils for spicy cooking in which the absence of olive oil will be less noticeable. Continue to use a small amount of olive oil on salads, but use a blended oil containing only a small percent of olive oil as the

242

all-purpose oil. Or he can blend his own mixture using a small amount of olive oil with one of the polyunsaturated oils.

I am a college student and notice sunflower seeds have become a real craze on campus. Are they good for you nutritionally, and how fattening are they?

Sunflower seeds, nutritionally fine, have become quite popular with the population at large. The seeds contain oil, protein, a good amount of iron, and some B vitamins.

They may be a nutritional hazard only to the dieter who consumes them in large quantities. Each tablespoon of kernels contains about 45 calories. A fairly small bag of kernels, weighing 5½ ounces, would supply 880 calories. That's quite a sizable snack.

Incidentally, sunflower seeds have begun to enjoy a wide market on the commercial level, too. In the past few years, there has been increasing interest in them. (Although sunflower is not a major oilseed crop in the United States, in world production it is second only to soybean oil.)

A natural question is: "What about sunflower oil on a cholesterol-lowering diet?" Interestingly enough, growing conditions affect the composition of the oil. Oil extracted from seeds grown in the north is much higher in polyunsaturates than that from seeds grown in the south. At present, most sunflower seeds grown for oil come from two northern states, Minnesota and North Dakota.

The meal left over after the oil is extracted contains good quality protein and is currently used in animal feed mixtures. And, once technological problems are ironed out, the meal might also provide us with another vegetable protein for human consumption.

You have mentioned submarine sandwiches as good food. While on vacation I ordered an Italian sub (or grinder) which arrived with two slices of bologna and lots of coleslaw. Surely this can't be what you had in mind?

It wasn't. I was talking about what we think of as the typical submarine sandwich, including meat and cheese as sources of protein, minerals and certain vitamins, some tomato for vitamin C, and some lettuce.

But bologna and coleslaw are not so bad. While maybe not as exciting to you as Italian ham and imported provolone cheese, the sandwich you were served gave you roughly the same protein and minerals, although the calcium from the cheese was lacking. And the coleslaw cabbage, if it hadn't been soaking and sitting around too long, probably was crisp and supplied some vitamin C.

Can cooking destroy vitamins and other nutrients? Can cooking add calories?

Yes to both questions. And cooking isn't the only treatment that can destroy nutrients. Many dreadful things can happen to food on the way to the table. Remember these rules: short storage, shortest possible cooking time, and least amount of cooking water. Also don't forget that crusty or well-browned baked goods have less thiamine; milk in glass containers can lose riboflavin unless kept out of the light and vitamin C is easily destroyed by heat.

Cooking can add calories. Frying can easily double them. But you can also cut calories by prudent cooking. Broiling meat, for example, decreases its fat content because the fat drips out and isn't eaten.

I've been trying to serve more fish in my house lately. Are some fish less fattening than others? Do you have any suggestions for preparing it, other than by broiling, that don't add too many extra calories?

There is considerable variability in the caloric value of fish. They divide mainly into two groups. There are about 115 calories in 4-ounce portions of "white" fish, such as halibut, perch, sea bass, haddock, cod and kingfish; flounder, one of the leanest, contains about 80 calories in 4 ounces. The fattier fish include salmon, mackerel and shad; a 4-ounce piece of one of these averages about 220 calories.

There are many ways to prepare fish other than to encase it beyond recognition in a coating of bread crumbs and then deep-fry it. Creative fish cookery, excellent in many foreign countries, unfortunately hasn't migrated to our shores.

Next time, for instance, try haddock *à l'Indienne:* Lightly brown two onions and clove of garlic in oil (polyunsaturated, of course). Transfer to a heat-proof dish. Place on the onions I pound of haddock fillets, sprinkle with parsley. Pour on a cup of dry white wine, 2½ tablespoons curry powder, and a pinch of thyme. Bake 10 minutes at 400° F. Then add ¾ cup yogurt, sprinkle with salt and pepper. Cook 10 minutes more. Serve with rice. That will be 200 calories per serving to each of four, 60 fewer than in 4 ounces of lean, broiled sirloin.

Fish need be neither uninteresting nor fattening!

Do you have some suggestions for making white fish a bit more exciting than just plain broiling?

Poaching is another good way to prepare not only fillets but fish steaks such as salmon or halibut. To poach fish, simmer it in fish stock or in a seasoned wine and water mixture for a short period of time.

It is uncommon for the American housewife to make fish stock, but it is really no more complicated than making chicken soup. Since it freezes well it can be made in amounts larger than those immediately needed and stored. The bones and fish trimmings used to make fish stock are generally yours for the asking at the fish store.

Poached fish can be served plain with lemon, or, if you can afford the calories, with a cream sauce made from the broth, some skim milk, polyunsaturated margarine and even a few mushrooms or some chopped shellfish, or both. A good basic cookbook can provide you with specific instructions for both the stock and the poached fish.

Getting back to the plain broiled fish for the moment. It need not be so plain. For variety, try serving it sprinkled with mushrooms, browned in a little oil, and a few toasted almonds, or with some chopped green peppers, onions and peeled tomatoes lightly browned in a trace of oil. Don't forget that leftover fish can be made into a very good salad for tomorrow's lunch.

I am a dieter who cannot stand dry salad. Can you suggest some low-calorie dressing ideas?

Many people look forward to the giant salad bowl dripping with Roquefort cheese dressing. But there are ways to enjoy salad without such 140-calories-a-tablespoon extravagance.

45

If you want to be a caloric conservative, one of the best methods is to use a seasoned wine vinegar. Add chopped onion, crushed garlic, dry mustard, salt and pepper, and herbs such as thyme and basil. You can also try tomato juice, Worcestershire sauce and chopped green pepper.

For a thicker dressing, cook the tomato juice with cornstarch before adding seasonings. Many people, even conscientious dieters, prefer to spend a few calories on salad dressing. One way is to make a standard vinegar and oil dressing, but change the ratio of vinegar to oil. The usual recipe calls for two or three parts oil to one of vinegar. By reversing a 2 to 1 recipe, you reduce the calories in a two-tablespoon serving from 160 to 80.

For a tasty dressing at 100 calories per two-tablespoon serving, use equal parts of mayonnaise and lemon juice seasoned with chives and capers. Yogurt also serves as a base for seasoning, and two tablespoons of plain yogurt contain only 20 calories.

My husband is on a cholesterol-lowering diet. He's lost quite a bit of weight. In fact, he really seems a little too thin. Can you suggest some desserts, besides fruit, which fall within the acceptable category?

There are a number of desserts that are quite acceptable for those lucky souls for whom excess weight is not a problem. Among commercially available cookies low in fat are raisin biscuits, ginger snaps, fig newtons and arrowroot cookies.

Custard may be prepared with two egg whites for each 1¼ cups of skim milk. Angel cake, made only with egg whites, is fine, too.

You can make chiffon cake from a mix, using only one egg and one egg white rather than the two the recipe suggests.

Pie crust made with corn, cottonseed or soybean oil is also acceptable.

Actually, the dessert possibilities are really limitless. The key to developing your own recipe file of desserts is, first, to substitute skim milk for whole. Then use oils or the acceptable margarines in place of butter and substitute two egg whites for each whole egg in a recipe. Or you might use two egg whites and only one egg, particularly if only a small portion is to be eaten at a meal, one serving out of a ten-serving cake, for example.

> *Since we have begun watching both our cholesterol and our food budget more closely, we're eating more turkey. My family prefers it stuffed, and they complain that stuffing cooked separately just doesn't taste the same. In warm weather I am particularly concerned about avoiding food poisoning. Can stuffed turkey be handled safely, even in the summer?*

Yes, it can. But before you give up on cooking it separately, try using chicken broth for the liquid in your stuffing. After all, the flavor your family likes comes from the juices produced during cooking. You might then like to fill the cavity with roughly chopped onions, celery, carrots and parsley, seasoned with salt and pepper and some herbs. The technique improves the flavor of the turkey itself.

If you do stick to the old method, three rules should keep your stuffing safe: First, stuff the bird just before roasting. Second, remove all the stuffing as soon as it is cooked. And third, refrigerate the leftovers promptly. Stuffing left inside the cavity and allowed to cool too gradually or left too long at room temperature can set the stage for food-borne infection.

> *My husband and I are quite fond of shad roe. When it's in season, in fact, we may eat it as often as twice a week. Is there any harm in this?*

Roe are eggs and all eggs, whether fish or fowl, are high in cholesterol. Therefore, you may want to cut down to once a week and limit yourself to not more than a 4-ounce serving.

Here's one method that's better, from both the viewpoints of taste and nutrition, than most for preparing roe: for four medium servings, heat 3 tablespoons oil in a heavy skillet; add 2 medium roe. Sprinkle with salt and pepper. Cook roe on both sides, turning once, about 12 minutes. When lightly brown, place on serving dish. Add to the pan 2 teaspoons lemon juice, 1 tablespoon chopped parsley, 2 teaspoons chopped chives, 1 teaspoon tarragon and a teaspoon of chervil. Pour over the roe

and serve.

I trust that my preface has made it clear that this book does not pretend to be the last word on nutrition. That book will never be written. You will agree, I believe, that I have offered no easy formulas, no quick solutions, no painless prescriptions. Instead, in these pages, I have attempted to provide a sane "diet for living," using the word "diet" in its primary sense:

> **diet**—Habitual course of living or, esp., feeding; hence, food and drink regularly provided or consumed; fare.
>
> —*Webster's New Collegiate Dictionary*

I have attempted to present my beliefs in an informal—even lighthearted—style, for I firmly believe that a good diet is not only one which will contribute to your good health but also one which should help maintain you in good cheer. The quest for a longer life certainly need not imply foregoing the pursuit of whatever happiness you and yours obtain at the dinner table.

Bon appétit!—but good appetite seasoned with understanding and common sense!

APPENDICES

APPENDIX ONE

What Can You Get for 100 Calories?

Food	*Amount*
Apple	1 large
Banana	1 medium
Beef, lean	2 ounces
Bread, whole wheat	2 thin slices
Butter	1 tablespoon
Cheese, cheddar	1 ounce
Cheese, cottage	½ cup
Chicken, light meat	2 ounces
Chocolate, sweet	2/3 ounce
Cola	8 ounces
Corn	1 large ear
Crackers, graham	4
Cream, heavy	2 tablespoons
Cream, light	3 tablespoons
French dressing	1 tablespoon
Grapefruit	1 medium
Haddock, fresh or frozen	3½ ounces

Ice cream, rich	¼ to 1/3 cup
Jam or jelly	2 tablespoons
Margarine	1 tablespoon
Mayonnaise	1 tablespoon
Milk, skim	1¼ cups
Milk, whole	¾ cup
Orange juice	1 cup
Peanut butter	1 tablespoon
Potato, boiled	1 large
Saltines	8
Spinach, boiled	3 cups
Sugar	2 tablespoons
Tuna, oil pack	2 ounces
Tuna, water pack	3 ounces

APPENDIX TWO

Protein Content of Some Common Foods

Food	Serving	Protein in Grams	Protein Quality
Bread, wheat	1 slice	2–3	incomplete
Cereals	½ cup	1–3	incomplete
Cheese			
cottage	2 ounces	10	complete
cheddar	1 ounce	7	complete
Dried beans or peas	½ cup, cooked	7–8	incomplete
Egg	1 whole	6	complete
Fish	3 ounces	15–25	complete
Fruits	½ cup	1–2	incomplete
Meat	3 ounces	15–25	complete
Milk, whole or skim	1 cup	9	complete
Pasta	½ cup	2	incomplete
Peanut butter	1 tablespoon	4	incomplete

Poultry	3 ounces	15–25	complete
Rice	½ cup	2	incomplete
Vegetables	½ cup	1–3	incomplete

The reader should note that while the protein foods labeled "incomplete" do not, by themselves, have the right proportions of essential amino acids for human needs, a protein dish of excellent quality can be obtained simply by adding small amounts of milk, cheese, fish, or meat to such a mixture of "incomplete" plant proteins as, for example, rice and beans.

APPENDIX THREE

Fat and Cholesterol Content of Some Common Foods

Food	Serving	Cholesterol Milligrams (approx.)	Total Fat Grams	Type of Fat*
Butter	1 tablespoon	37	12	saturated
Cheese				
cheddar	1 ounce	30	9	saturated
cottage, creamed	1 ounce	4	1	saturated
Chicken	3 ounces	60	3	unsaturated
Egg	1	275	6	saturated
Fish, white	3 ounces	65	0.24	polyunsaturated
Margarine, soft	1 tablespoon	0	12	polyunsaturated

*The dominant type. Butter, for example, is predominantly a *saturated* fat. However, it has some unsaturated fatty acids and even a small amount of the polyunsaturates. Corn oil, on the other hand, has exactly the reverse: it is predominately *polyunsaturated,* with some unsaturates, and a small amount of saturated fat. Olive oil is predominately *unsaturated.*

Meat				
beef	3 ounces	70	16	saturated
lamb	3 ounces	65	16	saturated
liver	3 ounces	300	9	saturated
pork	3 ounces	60	24	saturated
Milk, whole	2 cups	25	18	saturated
Oils				
coconut	1 tablespoon	0	14	saturated
peanut	1 tablespoon	0	14	unsaturated
olive	1 tablespoon	0	14	unsaturated
corn	1 tablespoon	0	14	polyunsaturated
safflower	1 tablespoon	0	14	polyunsaturated
soybean	1 tablespoon	0	14	polyunsaturated
Oysters	3 ounces	200	1.5	polyunsaturated
Shrimp	3 ounces	125	0.6	polyunsaturated

APPENDIX FOUR

Carbohydrate Content of Some Common Foods

Food	Serving	Carbohydrate in grams	Nutrient Quality* of Food
Bread			
white, unenriched	1 slice	13	poor
white, enriched	1 slice	13	good
whole-grain	1 slice	13	excellent
Cereal			
bran flakes	1 cup	28	good
corn flakes, sugared	1 cup	36	poor
oatmeal	1 cup	23	excellent
Chocolate	1 ounce	14	poor
Dried beans or peas	½ cup	17–26	excellent
Flour			
white, enriched	2 tablespoons	11	good

*The nutrient quality is determined by the number of other nutrients associated with the carbohydrate. The complex carbohydrate in whole grains or legumes, for example, brings to the diet protein, essential fatty acids, vitamins and a number of minerals, as well as calories. Sugar and syrups, on the other hand, provide only empty calories.

whole grain	2 tablespoons	11	excellent
Fruits			
dried prunes	4	18	excellent
fresh orange	1	16	excellent
Milk	1 cup	12	excellent
Nuts	¼ cup	4–10	good
Pasta, enriched	½ cup	16	good
Potatoes	1	18	excellent
Rice, brown or enriched	½ cup	25	good
Soft drinks	8 oz.	21–33	none
Sugars	1 tablespoon	11	none
Syrups (molasses, honey)	1 tablespoon	13	poor
Vegetables			
green beans	½ cup	4	excellent
green peas	½ cup	10	excellent

APPENDIX
FIVE

The Vitamins and Minerals: What they do for us, what they do to us, and where we get them

I. The Fat-Soluble Vitamins—all stored in the body, so toxicity can be built up.

The Vitamin	Its Functions	The Effects of Too Little or Too Much	Where to Find It
A	Formation of normal skin and mucosa (the internal skin), bone and tooth formation, night and color vision.	*Deficiency:* deterioration of skin and mucosa, faulty bone and tooth development, deterioration of eyes, night blindness, blindness. *Excess:* drying and peeling of skin, loss of hair, bone and joint pain, fragile bones, enlarged liver and spleen, death.	Liver, butter and fortified margarine, cream, whole milk and cheese made from whole milk, carrots, dark green leafy vegetables.
D	Regulates intestinal absorption of calcium and phosphorus and the normal utilization of these minerals in bones and soft tissues; has a part in protein metabolism.	*Deficiency:* in children, delayed tooth development, large joints, soft bones easily deformed and broken, deformities of chest, skull, spine, and pelvis (rickets). In adults, osteomalacia (adult rickets) characterized by softening of bones. *Excess:* weakness, weight loss, vomiting, diarrhea, calcium deposits in soft tissues, kidney damage, death.	Direct exposure of skin to sunlight, fortified milk, fish-liver oils, small amounts are in summer butter, liver, egg yolk, and fatty fish like sardines, salmon, and tuna.

	Its Functions	The Effects of Too Little or Too Much	Where to Find It
E	Acts as an antioxidant to reduce oxidation of vitamin A, the carotenes, and polyunsaturated fatty acids.	*Deficiency:* (a deficiency is rare and difficult to cause experimentally) mild anemia and destruction of red blood cells. *Excess:* no conclusive evidence. Muscle damage and fatigue are among the suggestions.	Vegetable oils: cottonseed, safflower, sunflower, soybean; corn, almonds, peanuts, wheat germ, rice germ, asparagus, green leafy vegetables, liver, margarine, vegetable shortening.
K	Necessary for proper blood clotting.	*Deficiency:* prolonged clotting time, hemorrhagic disease in newborn infants. *Excess:* menaquinone, a synthetic form, has caused jaundice in newborn infants. Natural forms do not seem toxic. An excess in adults is unlikely.	Main source is synthesis by normal bacteria in the intestine. Foods: lettuce, spinach, kale, cauliflower, cabbage, other green leafy vegetables, liver, egg yolk, soybean oil.

II. The Water-Soluble Vitamins—not stored in the body. Large doses may act pharmacologically (as drugs).

The Vitamin	*Its Functions*	*The Effects of Too Little or Too Much*	*Where to Find It*
C (Ascorbic Acid)	Formation of collagen, the connective tissue of skin, tendons, and bone, formation of	*Deficiency:* poor bone and tooth development, bleeding gums, weakened cartilage and capillary walls, skin hemorrhages, anemia (scurvy). *Excess:* perhaps causes destruction of B_{12} in in-	Citrus fruits, tomatoes, cantaloupe and other melons, berries, green leafy vegetables, peppers, broccoli, cauliflower, fresh potatoes.

Vitamin	Function	Deficiency / Excess	Sources
	hemoglobin, absorption and use of iron, and possibly utilization (metabolism) of protein and carbohydrates. Conversion of folic acid to folinic acid, an active form.	gested food; may cause increased risk of renal calculi.	
B_1 (Thiamine)	Necessary for carbohydrate metabolism.	*Deficiency:* apathy, depression, poor appetite, lack of tone in the gastrointestinal tract, constipation, heart failure (beriberi). *Excess:* no known effect.	Whole-grain flours and cereals, wheat germ, seeds like sunflower and sesame, nuts like peanuts and pine nuts, legumes like soybeans, organ meats, pork, leafy vegetables.
B_2 (Riboflavin)	In enzymes that transport hydrogen in the body as part of the metab-	*Deficiency:* cracks at corners of lips, scaly skin around nose and ears, sore tongue and mouth, itching, burning eyes, sensitivity to light. *Excess:* no	Liver, kidney, cheese, milk, eggs, leafy vegetables, enriched bread, lean meat, beans and peas.

		known effect.	
	olism of carbohydrates, fat, and protein.		Organ meats, lean meats, poultry, fish, wheat germ and whole-grain flours and cereals, nuts, seeds, rice, beans and peas. The amino acid tryptophan can be converted to niacin in the body.
Niacin	Part of coenzymes necessary for hydrogen transportation and for health of all tissue cells.	*Deficiency:* skin rash, sore mouth and tongue, inflamed membranes in the digestive tract, bloody diarrhea, depression, mental disorientation, stupor (pellagra). *Excess:* flushing of skin, sometimes jaundice.	
B$_6$	Coenzyme especially involved in metabolism of protein. Essential for conversion of tryptophan to niacin.	*Deficiency:* dermatitis around eyes, at angles of mouth, sore mouth and smooth red tongue, weight loss, dizziness, vomiting, anemia, kidney stones, nervous disturbances and convulsions. *Excess:* no known effects.	Seeds like sunflower, wheat germ and bran, whole-grain bread, flours and cereals, liver, meats, fish, and poultry, potatoes, beans, brown rice.
Pantothenic Acid	Part of coenzyme A, which is essential to many chemical reactions in the body, particularly me-	*Deficiency:* unlikely, unless part of a deficiency of all B vitamins. Then symptoms include headache and fatigue, insomnia, abdominal distress, numb, tingling hands and feet, muscle cramps, loss of coordination and per-	Liver, eggs, wheat germ or bran, rice germ, peanuts, peas. Widely distributed in most foods. A deficiency seldom seen unless the diet consists of highly processed

	Function	Deficiency/Excess	Sources
	tabolism and release of energy from fat, protein, and carbohydrate.	sonality changes. *Excess:* no known effects.	foods, since processing results in large losses.
Biotin	Part of enzymes necessary for metabolism of protein, fat, and carbohydrate, energy release.	*Deficiency:* avidin, a protein in raw egg white, blocks biotin absorption. A deficiency is seen only when many raw egg whites are consumed over a long period. Then symptoms are dermatitis, loss of appetite, nausea, anemia, deep depression, insomnia, and muscle pain. *Excess:* no known effects.	Like pantothenic acid, biotin is widely distributed in foods. Liver, egg yolk, nuts, and legumes are especially good sources.
Folacin	Part of coenzymes that are essential for the synthesis of nucleic acids, vital to all cells.	*Deficiency:* smooth, red tongue, intestinal distress, diarrhea, macrocytic anemia, in which red blood cells are larger and fewer than normal, with less hemoglobin. Young red blood cells do not mature. *Excess:* no known effect.	Liver, leafy vegetables, dried beans and peas, green vegetables like asparagus and broccoli, nuts, fresh oranges, whole-wheat flours, breads, and cereals.
B_{12}	Coenzyme necessary for synthesis of nucleic acids and for synthesis	*Deficiency:* sore tongue, weakness, weight loss, tingling hands and feet, back pain, mental and nervous changes. Eventual result, often over a long pe-	B_{12} is only present in animal foods: liver, meats, poultry, fish and shellfish, eggs, and milk and milk products.

of at least one amino acid, aspartic acid.

riod of time, is pernicious anemia, in which new blood cells do not develop normally, and there is deterioration of the spinal cord that after a time becomes irreversible. A diet high in folacin can mask the hematologic (blood) symptoms of B_{12} deficiency, but does not prevent the neurologic (nerve) symptoms. *Excess:* no known effects.

III. *The Macro-Minerals*—those we need in larger amounts*

The Mineral	Its Functions	The Effects of Too Little or Too Much**	Where to Find It
Calcium	Necessary for hard bones and teeth, muscle contraction, especially normal heart rhythm, transmission of nerve impulses, proper blood clotting,	Deficiency: in children, stunted growth, retarded bone mineralization; poor bones and teeth, skeletal malformation (rickets). In adults, osteoporosis—brittle, porous bones resulting from demineralization. *Excess:* may contribute to kidney stones, high levels of calcium in blood and urine, and deposition in soft tissues.	Milk and hard cheeses, dark green leafy vegetables, small fish eaten with bones, soft cheeses, dried beans and peas, broccoli, artichokes, sesame seeds.

	Function	Deficiency	Sources
	and to activate a number of enzymes.		
Phosphorus	Necessary (with calcium) to form and strengthen bones, as part of the nucleic acids, and for metabolism of fats and carbohydrates.	*Deficiency:* seldom seen in humans eating a normal diet. Weakness, bone pain, loss of minerals, especially calcium, from bones, poor growth.	Organ meats, meat, fish, poultry, eggs, milk and cheese, nuts, beans and peas, whole grains.
Magnesium	Activates enzymes in carbohydrate metabolism and release of energy. Helps regulate body temperature, nerve and muscle contraction, and protein synthesis.	*Deficiency:* seen only in alcoholism, or in people on a diet limited to few, and highly processed, foods. Weakness, tremors, dizziness, spasms and convulsions, delirium and depression.	Whole grains, nuts, beans, green leafy vegetables. Processing may result in high losses of magnesium.

Sulfur	Part of proteins, especially in hair, nails, and cartilage, part of the B vitamins thiamine and biotin, takes part in detoxification reactions.	*Deficiency:* not found. A diet adequate in protein (several amino acids contain sulfur) will meet needs.	Eggs, meat, milk and cheese, nuts, legumes.
Sodium	Major constituent of fluid outside cells, regulates water balance, muscle contractions and nerve irritability.	*Deficiency:* rare. Nausea, diarrhea, abdominal and muscle cramps. *Excess:* probably a factor in inducing high blood pressure; certainly a low-sodium diet is essential in reducing blood pressure.	Salt, salted foods, MSG, soy sauce, baking powder, cheese, milk, shellfish, meat, fish, poultry, eggs.
Potassium	Major constituent of fluid inside cells. With sodium, regulation of water balance, nerve irritability and muscle contraction.	*Deficiency:* muscle weakness, nausea, depletion of glycogen, rapid heart beat, heart failure. *Excess:* not known.	Widely distributed in foods. Fruits, like dates, bananas, oranges, cantaloupe, tomatoes, vegetables, especially dark green leafy vegetables, liver, meat, fish, poultry, milk.

	traction, and heart rhythm. Necessary for protein synthesis and glucose formation.		
Chlorine	Part of the fluid outside the cells; takes part in the formation of gastric juice, absorption of vitamin B_{12} and iron; in stomach, suppresses growth of microorganisms in foods.	*Deficiency:* vomiting, diarrhea.	One-half of table salt (with sodium)

*The reader should keep in mind that research into the role of minerals in human nutrition is in about the same stage as research into the vitamins was in the early years of this century. What is listed above is only a brief summary of what we know, and don't know, in early 1975. Aluminum, arsenic, barium, bismuth, bromine, cadmium, germanium, gold, lead, lithium, mercury, rubidium, silver, strontium, titanium, and zirconium so far do not seem to have a role in nutrition—but who knows what discovery the next years may bring? This is one more reason why it is important to eat a varied, well-rounded diet of fresh or lightly processed foods, for many of the minerals, even those we do know to be essential, are removed in food processing and are not restored when the product is enriched.

**At very high levels, all elements can become toxic. The only "effects of excess" listed are those which may occur from faulty diets or excessive amounts of frequently prescribed supplements.

IV. The Trace Minerals† — those we need in small (sometimes almost infinitesimal) amounts

The Mineral	Its Functions	The Effects of Too Little or Too Much	Where to Find It
Iron	Transports and transfers oxygen in blood and tissues. Part of hemoglobin in blood, myoglobin in muscles, protoplasm of cells, cell nuclei, and many enzymes in tissues.	*Deficiency:* faulty digestion, changes in body levels of enzymes containing iron, cell damage, low iron stores, microcytic anemia (red cells smaller, level of hemoglobin in them is lower). *Excess:* skin pigmentation, lowered glucose tolerance, cirrhosis of the liver.	Liver, eggs, lean meats, dried beans and peas, nuts, dried fruits, whole grains, and green leafy vegetables.
Iodine	Vital constituent of the thyroid hormones, thyroxine and triiodothyronine, that regulate basal metabolism and influence growth, mental	*Deficiency:* goiter, and, if the mother has a severe iodine deficiency in the first three months of pregnancy or before conception, cretinism in infants. *Excess:* taken over an extended period, high levels depress thyroid activity, also causing goiter.	Iodized salt is the sure source, also seafood, vegetables *grown near the sea where soil is rich in iodine,* and butter, milk, cheese, and eggs *if the animal's ration has been rich in iodine.*

	Function	Deficiency / Excess	Sources
	development, and deposition of protein and fat in the body.		
Manganese	Part of many enzymes. Necessary to synthesize complex carbohydrates, fat, and cholesterol, to utilize glucose and fats, for muscle contraction, proper development of bones and the pancreas.	*Deficiency:* So far seen only in animals, with many different symptoms, among them sterility and abnormal fetuses, bone deformation, and muscle deformities.	Abundant in most foods, both plant and animal. Whole grains, legumes, and nuts are good sources.
Copper	Acts with iron to synthesize hemoglobin in red blood cells; necessary for glucose	*Deficiency:* in some infants fed cow's milk, inhibits hemoglobin formation, causing anemia. Deficiencies in adults are unknown. *Excess:* in Wilson's disease, a rather rare metabolic defect,	In most foods. Organ meats, shellfish, nuts, dried beans and peas, and cocoa are good sources. (Like iron, it is absent from dairy products.)

metabolism, formation of nerve walls and connective tissue.	there is abnormal storage in liver and other tissues, including eyes. Can result in uremia, heart defects, hypertension, and death if not treated.	
Zinc — Constituent of insulin and enzymes important to digestion, protein metabolism, and synthesis of nucleic acids.	*Deficiency:* (rare in the U.S.) retarded growth, even "dwarfism," retarded sexual development, anemia, poor wound healing. *Excess:* nausea, vomiting, diarrhea, fever.	Wheat germ and bran, whole grains, dried beans and peas, nuts, lean meats, fish, and poultry.
Fluorine — Normal component of teeth; necessary to prevent dental decay. May also be necessary with calcium and vitamin D to maintain strong bones and prevent demineralization in later life.	*Deficiency:* tooth decay in young children, possibly osteoporosis in adults. *Excess:* mottling of tooth enamel, deformed teeth and bones.	Water, either naturally or artificially fluoridated at a concentration of one part per million.

Chromium	Metabolism of glucose and protein, synthesis of fatty acids and cholesterol, insulin metabolism.	Deficiency: poor utilization of glucose, perhaps due to impaired insulin metabolism.	Corn oil, meats, whole grains.

†The trace minerals listed here are those we are sure are essential to man. Others that most probably are because we know them to be necessary for the higher animals are molybdenum, selenium, nickel, tin, vanadium, and silicon. We know that boron is necessary for plants and lower organisms.

APPENDIX
SIX

RECOMMENDED DAILY DIETARY ALLOWANCES,[a] Revised 1974

Designed for the maintenance of good nutrition of practically all healthy people in th[e] U.S.A.

	Age	Weight		Height		Energy	Protein	Fat-Soluble Vitamins Vitamin A Activity		Vitamin D	Vitamin E Activity[e]
	(years)	(kg)	(lbs)	(cm)	(in)	(kcal)[b]	(g)	(RE)[c]	(IU)	(IU)	(IU)
Infants	0.0–0.5	6	14	60	24	kg × 117	kg × 2.2	420[d]	1,400	400	4
	0.5–1.0	9	20	71	28	kg × 108	kg × 2.0	400	2,000	400	5
Children	1–3	13	28	86	34	1,300	23	400	2,000	400	7
	4–6	20	44	110	44	1,800	30	500	2,500	400	9
	7–10	30	66	135	54	2,400	36	700	3,300	400	10
Males	11–14	44	97	158	63	2,800	44	1,000	5,000	400	12
	15–18	61	134	172	69	3,000	54	1,000	5,000	400	15
	19–22	67	147	172	69	3,000	54	1,000	5,000	400	15
	23–50	70	154	172	69	2,700	56	1,000	5,000	400	15
	51+	70	154	172	69	2,400	56	1,000	5,000	400	15
Females	11–14	44	97	155	62	2,400	44	800	4,000	400	12
	15–18	54	119	162	65	2,100	48	800	4,000	400	12
	19–22	58	128	162	65	2,100	46	800	4,000	400	12
	23–50	58	128	162	65	2,000	46	800	4,000	400	12
	51+	58	128	162	65	1,800	46	800	4,000	400	12
Pregnant						+300	+30	1,000	5,000	400	15
Lactating						+500	+20	1,200	6,000	400	15

SOURCE: Food and Nutrition Board, National Academy of Sciences–National Research Council.

[a] The allowances are intended to provide for individual variations among most normal persons as they liv[e] in the United States under usual environmental stresses. Diets should be based on a variety of common food[s] in order to provide other nutrients for which human requirements have been less well defined.

[b] Kilojoules (kJ) = 4.2 × kcal.

[c] Retinol equivalents.

[d] Assumed to be all as retinol in milk during the first six months of life. All subsequent intakes are assume[d] to be half as retinol and half as β-carotene when calculated from international units. A

Fola-cin[f] (µg)	Nia-cin[g] (mg)	Ribo-flavin (mg)	Thia-min (mg)	Vita-min B_6 (mg)	Vita-min B_{12} (µg)	Cal-cium (mg)	Phos-phorus (mg)	Iodine (µg)	Iron (mg)	Mag-nesium (mg)	Zi (m
50	5	0.4	0.3	0.3	0.3	360	240	35	10	60	3
50	8	0.6	0.5	0.4	0.3	540	400	45	15	70	5
100	9	0.8	0.7	0.6	1.0	800	800	60	15	150	10
200	12	1.1	0.9	0.9	1.5	800	800	80	10	200	10
300	16	1.2	1.2	1.2	2.0	800	800	110	10	250	10
400	18	1.5	1.4	1.6	3.0	1,200	1,200	130	18	350	15
400	20	1.8	1.5	2.0	3.0	1,200	1,200	150	18	400	15
400	20	1.8	1.5	2.0	3.0	800	800	140	10	350	15
400	18	1.6	1.4	2.0	3.0	800	800	130	10	350	15
400	16	1.5	1.2	2.0	3.0	800	800	110	10	350	15
400	16	1.3	1.2	1.6	3.0	1,200	1,200	115	18	300	15
400	14	1.4	1.1	2.0	3.0	1,200	1,200	115	18	300	15
400	14	1.4	1.1	2.0	3.0	800	800	100	18	300	15
400	13	1.2	1.0	2.0	3.0	800	800	100	18	300	15
400	12	1.1	1.0	2.0	3.0	800	800	80	10	300	15
800	+2	+0.3	+0.3	2.5	4.0	1,200	1,200	125	18 +[h]	450	20
600	+4	+0.5	+0.3	2.5	4.0	1,200	1,200	150	18	450	25

retinol equivalents, three fourths are as retinol and one fourth as β-carotene.
[e] Total vitamin E activity, estimated to be 80 percent as α-tocopherol and 20 percent other tocopherols.
text for variation in allowances.
[f] The folacin allowances refer to dietary sources as determined by *Lactobacillus casei* assay. Pure form folacin may be effective in doses less than one fourth of the recommended dietary allowance.
[g] Although allowances are expressed as niacin, it is recognized that on the average 1 mg of niacin is deriv from each 60 mg of dietary tryptophan.
[h] This increased requirement cannot be met by ordinary diets; therefore, the use of supplemental iro recommended.

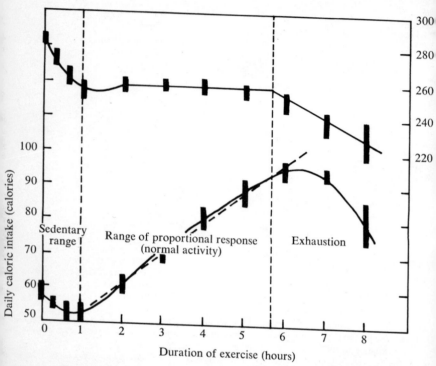

This graph is a summary of laboratory experiments with normal rats. You can see that their food intake do not necessarily increase with exercise. Rats exercised three or four hours a day eat more than those exercis for one hour, but they still maintain their body weight because of their activity. Our studies have shown th the same kind of graph can be drawn for humans. Within the wide range of normal activity, food inta will balance exercise, and weight will remain constant. At the level of physical exhaustion, food intake w diminish, in comparison to energy output, and weight will fall. In the sedentary range, where, alas, all t many adult Americans usually reside, food intake will not fall to match massive inactivity, and weight w rise. We are left with three choices in the matter of diet and exercise: we can remain inactive and mainta our weight by undereating, which is painful; we can resign ourselves and grow fat, which is disgraceful; we can exercise enough to eat normally and still maintain the right weight, which is inconvenient.

ENERGY EQUIVALENTS OF FOOD CALORIES EXPRESSED
IN MINUTES OF ACTIVITY*

Food	Calories	Walking[a]	Riding Bicycle[b]	Swimming[c]	Running[d]	Reclining
			Minutes of Activity			
Apple, large	101	19	12	9	5	78
Bacon, 2 strips	96	18	12	9	5	74
Banana, small	88	17	11	8	4	68
Beans, green, 1 c.	27	5	3	2	1	21
Beer, 1 glass	114	22	14	10	6	88
Bread and butter	78	15	10	7	4	60
Cake, 2-layer, 1/12	356	68	43	32	18	274
Carbonated beverage, 1 glass	106	20	13	9	5	82
Carrot, raw	42	8	5	4	2	32
Cereal, dry, 1/2 c. with milk, sugar	200	38	24	18	10	154
Cheese, cottage, 1 tbsp.	27	5	3	2	1	21
Cheese, Cheddar, 1 oz.	111	21	14	10	6	85
Chicken, fried, 1/2 breast	232	45	28	21	12	178
Chicken, TV dinner	542	104	66	48	28	417
Cookie, plain	15	3	2	1	1	12

Food	Calories	Minutes of Activity				
		Walking[a]	Riding Bicycle[b]	Swimming[c]	Running[d]	Reclining[e]
Cookie, chocolate chip	51	10	6	5	3	39
Doughnut	151	29	18	13	8	116
Egg, fried	110	21	13	10	6	85
Egg, boiled	77	15	9	7	4	59
French dressing, 1 tbsp.	59	11	7	5	3	45
Halibut steak, 1/4 lb.	205	39	25	18	11	158
Ham, 2 slices	167	32	20	15	9	128
Ice cream, 1/6 qt.	193	37	24	17	10	148
Ice cream soda	255	49	31	23	13	196
Ice milk, 1/6 qt.	144	28	18	13	7	111
Gelatin, with cream	117	23	14	10	6	90
Malted milk shake	502	97	61	45	26	386
Mayonnaise, 1 tbsp.	92	18	11	8	5	71
Milk, 1 glass	166	32	20	15	9	128
Milk, skim, 1 glass	81	16	10	7	4	62
Milk shake	421	81	51	38	22	324
Orange, medium	68	13	8	6	4	52
Orange juice, 1 glass	120	23	15	11	6	92
Pancake with syrup	124	24	15	11	6	95
Peach, medium	46	9	6	4	2	35
Peas, green, 1/2 c.	56	11	7	5	3	43
Pie, apple, 1/6	377	73	46	34	19	290
Pie, raisin, 1/6	437	84	53	39	23	336
Pizza, cheese, 1/8	180	35	22	16	9	138
Pork chop, loin	314	60	38	28	16	242
Potato chips, 1 serving	108	21	13	10	6	83
Sandwiches:						
Club	590	113	72	53	30	454
Hamburger	350	67	43	31	18	269
Roast beef with gravy	430	83	52	38	22	331
Tuna fish salad	278	53	34	25	14	214
Sherbet, 1/6 qt.	177	34	22	16	9	136
Shrimp, French fried	180	35	22	16	9	138
Spaghetti, 1 serving	396	76	48	35	20	305
Steak, T-bone	235	45	29	21	12	181
Strawberry shortcake	400	77	49	36	21	308

[a] Energy cost of walking for 150-lb. individual-5.2 calories per minute at 3.5 m.p.h.
[b] Energy cost of riding bicycle-8.2 calories per minute.
[c] Energy cost of swimming-11.2 calories per minute.
[d] Energy cost of running-19.4 calories per minute.
[e] Energy cost of reclining-1.3 calories per minute.

*From: Konishi, F. "Food energy equivalents of various activities," *J. Amer. Dietetic Assoc.*, 46 (1965), 186. Used by permission.

To convert

from	*to*	*multiply by*
centimeters	inches	.3937
cubic feet	cubic meters	.0283
feet	meters	.3048
gallons (U.S.)	liters	3.7853
inches	millimeters	25.4000
inches	centimeters	2.5400
kilograms	pounds (avoirdupois)	2.2046
liters	gallons (U.S.)	.2643
liters	pints (liquid)	2.1134
liters	quarts (dry)	.9081
liters	quarts (liquid)	1.0567
millimeters	inches	.0394
ounces	grams	28.3495
pounds (avoirdupois)	kilograms	.4536
quarts (dry)	liters	1.1012
quarts (liquid)	liters	.9463